SO-BBF-782

"This book comes at the perfect time. This is a guide for women and men, young and old, with tools for everyone—educators, policy makers, therapists, and anyone who wants to navigate oppressive patriarchy—to find specific ways to handle the workplace, health care, education, or deal with their own personal relationships. Everyone should read this book to heal and move forward, to create a new society, empowered and stronger for it."

—**Tammy Nelson, PhD**, director of the Integrative Sex Therapy Institute, TEDx speaker, and author of The New Monogamy

"The Feminist Handbook is not only chock-full of information, but also has activities that the reader can personalize for many of the major points. This guided, experiential focus will help the reader really incorporate various issues from a feminist perspective."

—**Judith Belmont, MS**, author of Embrace Your Greatness

"This unique book challenges you to change yourself in order make changes in the world around you. By integrating feminist scholarship with personal reflection and behavioral strategies, the reader will find ways to express their values and prioritize self-care. This is a must-read for those who want to express their voice and work for social justice, while nurturing themselves and their relationships in the process."

—**Sheela Raja, PhD**, associate professor and clinical psychologist at the University of Illinois at Chicago, author of Overcoming Trauma and PTSD, and coauthor of The PTSD Survival Guide for Teens and The Sexual Trauma Workbook for Teen Girls

"The Feminist Handbook is a must-read for anyone who wants to gain self-awareness and take action to improve the lives of women (and men). Joanne Bagshaw has given an important gift to the world—a powerful, accessible, and actionable guide to intersectional feminism."

—**Julie de Azevedo Hanks, PhD, LCSW**, author of The Assertiveness Guide for Women, owner of Wasatch Family Therapy, and assistant professor of social work at Utah Valley University

"In the times of #blacklivesmatter, #metoo, and #timesup, Joanne Bagshaw gives us a gift where we can deeply explore the connections of intersectional feminism to our lived experiences. Patriarchy has long outlived itself, and Bagshaw provides step-by-step learning for how to resist, engage in body liberation, and work for sexual and reproductive justice."

—**Anneliese Singh, PhD, LPC**, professor and associate dean of diversity, equity, and inclusion at the University of Georgia; and author of The Racial Healing Handbook and The Queer and Transgender Resilience Workbook

The Social Justice Handbook Series

As culture evolves, we need new tools to help us cope and interact with our social world in ways that feel authentic and empowered. That's why New Harbinger created the *Social Justice Handbook* series—a series that teaches readers how to use practical, psychology-based tools to challenge and transform dominant culture, both in their daily lives and in their communities.

Written by thought leaders in the fields of psychology, sociology, gender, and ethnic studies, the *Social Justice Handbook* series offers evidence-based strategies for coping with a broad range of social inequities that impact quality of life. As research has shown us, social oppression can lead to mental health issues such as depression, anxiety, trauma, lowered self-esteem, and self-harm. These handbooks provide accessible social analysis, as well as thoughtful activities and exercises based on the latest psychological methods to help readers unlearn internalized negative messages, resist social inequities, transform their communities, and challenge dominant culture to be equitable for all.

The handbooks also serve as a hands-on resource for therapists who wish to integrate an understanding and acknowledgement of how multiple social issues impact their clients to provide relevant and supportive care.

For a complete list of books in
the *Social Justice Handbook* series,
visit newharbinger.com.

THE FEMINIST HANDBOOK

Practical Tools *to*
Resist Sexism
and Dismantle
the Patriarchy

JOANNE L. BAGSHAW, PhD

New Harbinger Publications, Inc.

Publisher's Note

This publication is designed to provide accurate and authoritative information in regard to the subject matter covered. It is sold with the understanding that the publisher is not engaged in rendering psychological, financial, legal, or other professional services. If expert assistance or counseling is needed, the services of a competent professional should be sought.

Distributed in Canada by Raincoast Books

Copyright © 2019 by Joanne L. Bagshaw
    New Harbinger Publications, Inc.
    5674 Shattuck Avenue
    Oakland, CA 94609
    www.newharbinger.com

Cover design by Sara Christian

Acquired by Elizabeth Hollis Hansen

Edited by Brady Kahn

All Rights Reserved

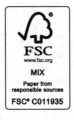 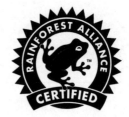

Library of Congress Cataloging-in-Publication Data on file

Printed in the United States of America

21   20   19

10 9 8 7 6 5 4 3 2 1   First Printing

For Ava, so that you may have a better, safer world to live in.

Contents

Contents

Foreword

One of the constant issues women face in leading healthier, happier lives is that we are not educated in ways that enable us to make sense of our experiences as women. Instead, we can find ourselves fighting against an enduring cultural hostility to any acknowledgment of our experiences and what they mean to us personally, professionally, and politically. In some cases this hostility is blunt. We see it in fractious political debates about wage gaps, pregnancy discrimination, or reproductive justice. More often, however, it's less visible, manifested in the subtle granularity of habits, traditions, and storytelling. It is baked into how we learn history and how we think about our religious, political, and media institutions, all of which are grounded in the idea that the men who rule and have the power to shape the world do so because they are "born to" instead of because others are systemically and violently oppressed. One of the most powerful constraints on women's equality remains how much of the nitty-gritty of our lives is still considered taboo or unwelcome in private and pubic conversation, not "family friendly" in media, and not centrally important to politics. Women and people who are feminine continue to be harmed by the centering of men and masculinity, which are the pillars of patriarchal social organization. In other words, we are harmed because we live in a patriarchal world optimized to silence us.

For many years I've studied, written, and talked about this world and the role that feminism plays in understanding and challenging it. During that time, three issues have remained constant and primary for the women and men with whom I've come in contact. First, why does it often take us, as individuals, so long to learn about and understand what feminism is, its urgency and importance? Second, what can we do, as individuals and as a society, to unlearn damaging lessons and to further the aims of feminism? And third, how do we cultivate genuinely egalitarian beliefs, mores, and values earlier, so that this unlearning is no longer necessary? These questions result from the conditions of patriarchy itself: a systemic and intersectional oppression of women that dictates how we live and what roles we play in our interpersonal relationships, our schools, our places of worship, and our governance.

These questions are grounded in our early childhood socialization and education. It is as children that most of us learn to narrowly define gender as binary and oppositional and then, almost always, to disdain femininity in anyone. It is as children that girls learn to adapt in silence to subtle and often socially tolerated and institutionally perpetuated discrimination. As we grow up, we are taught to ignore, work around, and minimize the blunt threat and reality of the violence that surrounds us, whether in our homes or on public streets. It is rare for a woman to reach adulthood with any real and useful knowledge about the confusion, stress, pain, and trauma that can be associated with having (or *not* having) a body that conforms to roles and ideals, a body that menstruates, gestates, and gives birth (or doesn't). While we all experience discrimination and oppression differently and in different measure, and, indeed, can often oppress others, we share the understanding that shrouding ourselves in shame is preferable to demanding respect, trust, and power. As a result, women often struggle—from cradle to grave—with saying what we feel and need; we struggle to demand care, fairness, respect, and our rights.

It is often the case that we come to feminism reluctantly and with little or no understanding of the diversities of feminism or with the history of liberation movements, or with the ways in which both shape our lives every day. Instead we learn, as children, to fold the tremendous costs of patriarchy into ourselves. We grow into adults who live, ultimately, maladaptively.

This book provides the words, tools, and practical guidelines necessary to unlearn these powerful, pervasive, and limiting lessons.

Feminism, as Joanne Bagshaw eloquently and succinctly explains, is the antidote to the harms and predations of patriarchy and its multiple, intersecting oppressions. This book is written so that readers can cultivate resilient and healthy ways of living feminist lives. Joanne begins with one of the clearest and most concise explanations of feminism, patriarchy, and privilege that you will ever read. Throughout the book, she provides a necessary language along with specific, practical tools and strategies for thinking about and living a feminist life.

The Feminist Handbook is an invaluable contribution. It answers the most urgent question of all: how do we make sense of the world in a way that helps instead of hurts women? The starting point, as this book illustrates so compellingly, is to understand feminism's most basic and fundamental unit: the ability to tell the truth about your life without fear or shame and with dignity and compassion—for yourself and for others. It is a simple step that anyone can take, and it can, as she shows us here, be lifesaving.

—Soraya Chemaly
Writer and journalist

PART 1

LEARNING THE LANGUAGE

CHAPTER ONE

Patriarchy, Privilege, and Oppression

"…feminism is the only ongoing conversation about patriarchy that can lead to a way out."

—Allan G. Johnson, *The Gender Knot*

Stephanie is an executive at her company. She is known as a hard worker, with stellar performance reviews since she began working at this company five years ago. One day, Stephanie happily came to work to announce to her colleagues, and her boss, that she is three months pregnant. A few days later, after a lunchtime celebration with cake and balloons, her boss pulled her aside and said: "I was considering you for a promotion, but now I'm not so sure you're the right person for that job, as it requires extra hours and some travel. But congratulations. I guess you're on the mommy track now." Stephanie was devastated. She has worked hard and planned the right time to have a child. She is financially secure, with a supportive partner who works flexible hours. She has family nearby who are willing and able to help with childcare too. Stephanie planned on taking maternity leave and returning to work full-time afterward at this same company, doing the work that she loves, and she was hopeful and excited about the possibility of being promoted. But now she's unsure. Is having a child going to impact her career? Should it? Stephanie begins to second-guess her choices and options now. If she were to leave this company and go to another, would she make the same salary? Would anyone hire her while she's pregnant? How stressful would it be to start a new job where she would have to prove herself all over again, but this time with a new baby? Stephanie feels limited and resigned to accept what appears to be a path that she didn't plan for: the mommy track.

Discrimination against pregnant women has been illegal since 1978, when Congress passed the Pregnancy Discrimination Act. The Pregnancy Discrimination Act is an amendment to the Civil Rights Act of 1964, and demands that women who are "affected by pregnancy, childbirth or related medical conditions…be treated the same for all employment-related purposes…" So how could Stephanie's manager overlook her for a promotion if discrimination against pregnant women is illegal?

Although Stephanie's company proudly displays their antidiscrimination statement and policies on their website, in practice, some managers hold perceptions and assumptions about working mothers that can hold back women like Stephanie from moving ahead with their career while raising children. Stephanie would likely have a hard time proving discrimination in this case if she were to consider a lawsuit, because no one overheard the conversation and because other women have been promoted in her department, most notably her manager, who is a working mother with three college-aged children. Stephanie is right to be concerned. Although the law protects her, women in all industries, and women of all races and classes, experience pregnancy discrimination. For instance, according to the National Partnership for Women and Families (2016), between the years 2011 and 2015, almost 31,000 charges of pregnancy discrimination were filed with the US Equal Employment Opportunity Commission (EEOC).

Discrimination that is clearly illegal still occurs because oppression and discrimination are supported by a patriarchal system.

THE PATRIARCHY IS A SYSTEM

The patriarchy is not about individual men. It is a social system that *we all* participate in, which is male-identified and promotes male privilege. Our culture demonstrates a patriarchal system in the ways described next (Johnson 2014). Following each example are some questions to help you reflect on your experience of living in a patriarchy.

Who Possesses Authority?

Positions of authority—including political leaders, heads of state, and religious, military, and educational leaders—are typically held by men. Women do hold these positions sometimes, but not as often as men, and when they are in these positions, women are often expected to act in ways that are typically considered masculine and then are likely to be called "bossy" or "a bitch" as a result and also likely to be seen as less attractive (Eagly and Carli 2007). As a society, we tend to equate leadership with masculinity.

- When you express leadership skills, how do others react to you?

- Are there times when you would like to be a leader but don't exert the effort? What holds you back?

What Does Our Society Value Most?

Most of our cultural ideas about what is normal, good, and important are associated with men and masculinity. Have you noticed how the pronoun "he" is used as a default? Additionally, our society's core values of autonomy and toughness, and its high regard for competition, are based on our ideas of what masculinity is.

- Do you find that traditional values of masculinity, as described above, reflect you and your values? Do they reflect everyone's values? Whose values are being represented?

- Masculine values aren't inherently wrong or bad, but alone, they are limiting. What values are missing from our society's core value system?

Who's the Main Subject?

Our culture is centered on men. For example, most Hollywood movies revolve around men's lives and men's stories. Even movies that are created for a female audience and have female leads contain more dialogue between men than between women (Anderson and Daniels 2016).

- Think about the last film you saw. Compare the male and female characters and what they were doing in the film. What differences did you notice?

- When you ask a male friend or partner to see a film with you whose lead actors are women, what is their response? How does their response make you feel?

Who's Expected to Be in Control?

It is a cultural standard for men to remain in control at all times. Men are expected to be unemotional, strong, and independent, and women are expected to be the opposite. Men are also expected to be in control of situations, able to take charge and lead any situation if necessary. Control is essential to patriarchy, because our culture assumes the superiority of the group that maintains control. The cultural belief that men are entitled to be in control because they earned it is how men maintain their privilege in a patriarchal society (Johnson 2014).

- Can you think of an experience where a man was not in control? How was he regarded? What names was he called?

- Can you recall an experience where a woman was in control of a man? How was she regarded? What names was she called?

- We'll explore the concept of privilege next, but first let's reflect on what patriarchy is, and why this is the place to start exploring feminism.

FEMINISM AS AN ANTIDOTE TO PATRIARCHY

As a society, we have participated in creating a structure that supports the superiority of men over women. We have done this by creating an image of masculinity that is associated with power, control, status, leadership, independence, competition, and domination. To counteract the negative effects of sexism and discrimination that are the outgrowth of living within a patriarchal society, we need to create a different structure that rejects hierarchy and superiority and instead promotes equality for everyone.

Feminism isn't about women being equal to men. Feminism means liberation from patriarchal values and structures that are oppressive to all of us. Within a patriarchy, men are the blueprint, but because a patriarchy is also a hierarchy, categories of difference separate us. In simplistic terms, where you identify in this hierarchy will affect your value in society and your access to resources ranging from jobs to your physical safety in the world.

ACTIVITY: How Are You Different?

Check off any categories of difference that you identify with in this list:

- ☐ You are a member of the LGBTQIA community.

- ☐ You are a person of color.

- ☐ You are a member of the lower middle class, working class, or have low income or are poor.

- ☐ You are a member of any religion other than Christian.

- ☐ You do not have a college education.

☐ You are an immigrant.

☐ English is not your first language.

☐ You are indigenous.

☐ You are disabled.

☐ You are an older adult.

These categories represent areas where you may differ from the patriarchal blueprint. You may recognize these areas of difference as places where you don't benefit from a patriarchal hierarchy.

Feminism is the antidote to patriarchy, because the goal of feminism is to create liberation from hierarchical oppressive structures for everyone. Before we begin dismantling the patriarchy, however, let's explore what privilege is and its relationship to the patriarchy.

Privilege

The patriarchy is a social system that is centered around *privilege*, which simply means having unearned advantages and access to resources. For example, being an American citizen is a privilege in comparison to others who live in the developing world. An individual born in the United States didn't necessarily do anything other than being born to have the right to live here, travel abroad and return at will, or be protected by the Constitution.

Having privilege doesn't mean that you are rich, have had an easy life, or that you haven't struggled. It means that you have advantages. You've been treated a certain way, and can expect to be treated a certain way, that is different from how others are treated. The more privilege you have, the more resources and advantages you have access to, which gives you more power in society and protection from experiencing certain social problems, because you have more choices. Privileged people tend to be part of the dominant group in society and are seen as superior. And when privileged people have institutional power and prejudice, they are able to push less privileged people to the margins of society by denying access to resources. We'll discuss institutional power more later in the chapter.

Let's compare the life experiences of two white women to illustrate the ways privilege can give one woman advantages over another:

Erica is a thirty-two-year-old white heterosexual married woman. She and her husband own a home in a suburban neighborhood with good public schools that their two children attend.

Erica's children are in elementary school, and she works from home part-time doing some freelance writing while they are in school and on the weekends when her husband is home to help with the kids. Erica's husband is a professional with a graduate degree. He has a good income, and his parents paid for his college, so he doesn't have any student loan debt. Erica put herself through college while working part-time and has some small student loans, but when her grandmother passed away, she left Erica a modest inheritance that helped Erica and her husband purchase their first home. Erica and her husband aren't wealthy, but they live a comfortable, upper middle-class life.

Claudia is a twenty-three-year-old white heterosexual single mother living with her young son, Wyatt, and her mother. Claudia has a high school education and works as a waitress in the evening and weekends. During the day she takes care of her mother, who has numerous health issues and is on disability. Claudia's father died several years ago. Neither of her parents went to college, and they were low income. Claudia did not consider college after graduating from high school, as she didn't think it was financially feasible, plus no one in her family had gone to college, and at the time she didn't see the value in furthering her education. Now Claudia hopes to attend the local community college as a nursing student, once Wyatt gets a little older and is in school. Claudia's local public school system is okay but not great. Claudia wishes she could send Wyatt to a private school but can't afford it. She's considering home schooling him but doesn't know how she could manage doing that along with taking care of her mother and having a work schedule that changes from week to week. Claudia rents the house they live in and dreams that someday she will be able to own her home.

Both women in these vignettes have some privilege because they are white and heterosexual, which makes them members of two dominant groups in our society. Erica is married, which gives her a higher social status than Claudia, plus she reaps several benefits of having a partner whose income helps support her to stay at home with her children. Erica's husband financed his college education, which probably helped him gain a higher salaried job, allowing them to live in a good school district, and Erica's inherited money went toward buying a house. Claudia, on the other hand, is a young single parent with no college education and without a steady income, who takes care of her disabled mother. Claudia grew up lower income, and even now as a young adult and mother, she has access to fewer resources and choices. It's easy to see where Claudia is challenged in life, but it may be hard to see her privilege at first, because privilege is often invisible. The key to understanding the invisibility of privilege is to consider the role that systemic oppression plays in maintaining privilege, and from there, you can see how Claudia has more opportunities because of her race.

ACTIVITY: Your Challenges and Advantages

Take a moment to reflect on a challenge that you have experienced or are experiencing in your life. In what ways has this experience been challenging to you, based on your identity? And in what ways might you have some advantages that have helped you, or at least made this challenge somewhat easier for you, compared to if you did not have these advantages?

Challenges	Advantages

Systemic Oppression

If Claudia were African-American or a Latina, her situation would be far more challenging. Historic policies such as slavery, Jim Crow, and school segregation, and mass incarceration today are examples of *structural inequities* that create *systemic oppression*, making day-to-day life more difficult for African-Americans as a group than for whites (Hanks, Solomon, and Weller 2018). African-Americans and Latinx household wealth is far below the wealth of white families, and both African-American and Latina women are paid less than white women (Hegewisch and Williams-Baron 2018). This comes from the fact that African-American families on average have less access to stable jobs and decent wages than their neighbors (Copeland 2014).

Let's look briefly at the issue of mass incarceration to illustrate how a social issue is created by our educational system and school policies within this institution. Mass incarceration begins as early as preschool in the school-to-prison pipeline. Black and Latinx children are suspended and expelled from school at much higher rates than their white peers. As early as preschool, black children, particularly boys, comprise 48 percent of young children who are expelled from school, despite research that shows that black children aren't any more disruptive than children of other races (Flannery 2015). Expelled students are more likely to drop out of school and wind up in the juvenile justice system and later in prison (Flannery 2014). Systemic oppression like mass incarceration reinforces beliefs and biases about social groups, which helps to maintain oppression and inequality.

The Nuances of Privilege

In a patriarchal society, men generally hold structural and institutional power. Structural and social institutions include government, law, medicine, and the media, and leadership positions within these institutions are primarily held by men. In early 2018, nearly 80 percent of the US Senate and House of Representatives was composed of men (CAWP 2018). The 2018 midterm elections added more than one hundred women to Congress, which was a historic feminist victory, particularly because the women elected were primarily women of color and represented religious minority groups and LGBTQIA women. However, the total percentage of women representatives in Congress is still only about 24 percent. The low percentage of females in Congress means that men—and mostly white men—are in the majority, making decisions that impact all of our lives.

But not all men have institutional power or access to racial privilege. Men who are members of marginalized social groups experience both oppression and privilege. A young man who is a high school graduate with a blue-collar job has less privilege than a middle-aged man with a professional degree and a white-collar job. African-American men may have some advantages as men, but do not have racial privilege. A transgender male experiences oppression and less privilege than a *cis-gender* male (whose gender identity and sex assigned at birth match) but may also experience advantages as a male. For instance, transgender men who have transitioned from female to male may experience more respect and authority at work than they did when they identified as female, in the same place of employment and position (Schilt 2006).

Privileged and Marginalized Groups

Privilege and oppression are simply about power dynamics. When some groups in society hold more power, naturally there will be groups who hold less. The groups with less power tend to be pushed to the margins of society, and the groups with power have more influence over those who have less. Privileged groups create the laws and policies and set the norms in society and are considered the baseline against which less privileged groups are compared (Goodman 2015).

Consider the US Congress again. When the majority of our political leaders, who are white males, make decisions based on a bias that centers around a white male perspective, those decisions don't necessarily reflect the wants and needs of their constituents and instead can enforce oppression. In 2017, a committee of thirty male Republican senators met to make decisions on a proposed health care bill and specifically discussed women's health care needs, and whether or not the bill should mandate prenatal care, maternity services, and screening for diseases like breast or cervical cancer as "essential benefits." Their plan, if passed, would have cut funding for many reproductive health care services that would impact women, particularly low-income women, so that many would have to go without health care, which is a form of oppression. Regardless of political affiliation, a roomful of men should not make decisions about women's health care. When privileged groups exercise their social power and decision making, they reinforce their biases, which manifests as oppression to marginalized groups in society (Goodman 2015).

Following are some examples of dominant and marginalized groups in our society.

Dominant Group	Marginalized Group
White	Latina, Asian-American, African-American, indigenous
Heterosexual	Bisexual, lesbian, gay, queer, intersex
American citizen	Noncitizen, immigrant, undocumented people

Dominant Group	Marginalized Group
Christian	Muslims, Jews, atheists
Upper class	Lower class, working class, blue collar, middle class
Middle-aged	Child, teenager, older adult
Able-bodied	Disabled, emotional or psychological disability
Cis-gender	Transgender, gender nonconforming

You most likely belong to some groups that are dominant and to others that are marginalized, because we are all three-dimensional beings with many identities.

ACTIVITY: What Social Groups Do You Identify With?

Make a list of the social groups that you belong to, based on the preceding chart.

_____

_____

_____

Are there social groups that you feel more comfortable identifying with? Are there social groups that are more difficult for you to identify with? Describe why you feel more comfortable identifying with some groups than others.

_____

_____

_____

_____

The following examples of privilege are based on Peggy McIntosh's (1989, 2010) work on identifying her personal experience with white privilege. Check off any of the examples below that apply to you. There's also space for you to add your own autobiographical examples of privilege that may not be listed here:

- ☐ Mainstream media represents you. For example, you can turn on any network, and find shows with people who look like you and represent your lifestyle.

- ☐ You are able to purchase cosmetics and products that match your skin tone without going to a specialty store. For example, the tone "nude" or "flesh colored" matches your skin color.

- ☐ Your religious holidays are recognized by your community with schools and government buildings closed.

- ☐ You do not have to hide your relationship with your partner.

- ☐ You are physically able to enter any building, park, or public bathroom.

- ☐ You are rarely asked where you are from.

- ☐ You do not have to prepare your child on how to deal with discrimination.

- ☐ You can opt out of worrying about some social problems, because they won't affect you personally.

- ☐ You are not afraid to call the police.

- ☐ Going to college was/is an expectation in your family.

- ☐ You have gone to the doctor for checkups.

- ☐ Politicians who make decisions and laws about your rights and health care are the same gender as you.

- ☐ You've never been told by a stranger to smile.

- ☐ You're not the punch line for jokes about age.

- ☐ Your identity is not considered a psychological disorder.

- ☐ _____

- ☐ _____

Understanding who has privilege can feel confusing or complicated because you may experience privilege in one category but not in another. For example, white women have privilege but not as much as white men, who have more *institutional power* than white women. Institutional power gives social groups the ability to decide what's right for others, decide who needs resources, and who will get resources.

You may also have difficulty identifying with having any privilege, particularly if you are a person of color who experiences multiple avenues of oppression (such as African-American, queer, and disabled), but still experience privilege as a Christian American citizen, for example. Having privilege in one area of your life doesn't necessarily protect you from oppression in other areas.

ACTIVITY: Explore the Nuances of Your Own Privilege

Reflect on your experience identifying with both dominant and marginalized groups. What does privilege and oppression look like in your life? How does the nuance of your own experience impact you?

_____

_____

_____

_____

_____

_____

By now you should have an understanding that the patriarchy is oppressive and not just toward women. Having or not having privilege isn't something you should be ashamed of or feel guilty about. However, the task of feminism is to dismantle patriarchy, which includes undoing other systems of hierarchy and oppression, like racism, which make privilege possible. Dismantling a system that privileges some but not others may seem like a daunting task, because quite frankly, it is. The place to start is to be willing to look honestly at yourself and reflect on your own privilege, particularly if you benefit from white privilege.

MAKING PRIVILEGE VISIBLE

Privilege thrives in a patriarchal society when it remains invisible and when you remain in denial. A key component in dismantling the patriarchy is recognizing privilege when you see it or experience it and finding ways to not participate in the patriarchal system and to stand up for others who are oppressed. Your first step in making privilege visible is to identify where in your life you are privileged, as you explored above, and to reflect honestly on how you benefit from privilege and how your actions (or inaction) may contribute to the oppression of other groups as well as to the patriarchy. Nonjudgmental mindfulness is a tool that can help you reflect on and connect with the places in your life where you experience privilege.

ACTIVITY: Use Nonjudgmental Mindfulness

Spend a moment reading all of the steps below before you practice this exercise.

1. Find a quiet place and time to spend reflecting on privilege and oppression.

2. Spend a few minutes focusing on your breathing. Notice your breath as you inhale and as you exhale. Don't try to change your breathing; act as an observer.

3. Accept your thoughts as they come, keeping your mind open, with curiosity. Come back to your breath if your mind wanders or if your thoughts begin to overwhelm you.

4. Allow yourself to visualize the ways that you benefit from privilege. Remember not to judge—simply accept the information with curiosity.

5. Allow yourself to visualize the ways that you don't experience privilege. If you find yourself having difficult emotions or self-judgmental thoughts, remember to come back to your breath and to remain curious about whatever information emerges.

6. Allow yourself to visualize the ways that your privilege might contribute to oppression. Keep practicing nonjudgmental curiosity.

7. Allow yourself to visualize the ways in which you might contribute to a patriarchal system.

Write down what you experienced during your meditation. Remember that the key part of the exercise is to not judge yourself but to remain open to and curious about your experience.

_____

_____

_____

_____

_____

_____

You can also break this meditation up into several different sessions if you want to focus more on different aspects of your privilege and contributions to oppression and patriarchy.

FEMINIST REFLECTION

Throughout this book, you will be exploring how you can develop your feminist identity. You've started by diving right into challenging topics like identifying the ways you are privileged and oppressed, and how you might contribute to the oppression of others. Understanding our own role in structures like patriarchy and oppression is not easy for anyone, so you are already off to a good start in developing your feminist identity. To deepen your exploration and understanding of feminism as you read this book, visit http://www.newharbinger.com/43805 to download a supplemental list of concepts covered in each chapter, along with suggested readings and discussion questions and activities. These resources will help you grow as a feminist and would also be suitable for a feminist book club.

The next chapter will look at how equality is fundamentally different for everyone. It will explore the history of the women's movement and what we need to change to make the feminist movement of today accessible to everyone.

CHAPTER TWO

It's Not Feminism
If It's Not Intersectional

"There is no such thing as a single-issue struggle, because we do not live single-issue lives."

—Audre Lorde

There are significant racial disparities between African-American and white women in terms of motherhood and infant mortality. African-American women are three to four times more likely to die from pregnancy-related causes than white women (Creanga et al. 2015; Callaghan 2012), and black infants have higher rates of infant mortality, due to low birth weight and preterm birth than white infants (Smith et al. 2018). Even when researchers control for risk factors like smoking or alcohol use, the disparity exists. The chronic stress that African-American women face because of the discrimination they experience in every aspect of their lives, even before they become pregnant, takes a toll on their bodies, threatening their life and the life of their babies (David and Collins 1991; Mustillo et al. 2004).

The high rates of motherhood mortality illustrate how race and gender intersect in the lives of African-American women. There's no one-size-fits-all brand of feminism. It's essential to give consideration to the ways that different systems of oppression affect women. The term *intersectionality* didn't always exist, but the need to understand different avenues of oppression and make feminism work for everyone has been present since the women's movement began in the nineteenth century.

WAVES OF FEMINISM

The feminist movement is best understood as happening in waves, representing peaks of activism spanning the nineteenth and twentieth centuries. Each wave focused on achieving specific goals of equality for women. The movement during the first and second waves was focused primarily on the rights of straight white middle-class women, leaving behind marginalized groups like LGBTQIA women, low-income women, and women of color. Third-wave feminists did a better job of celebrating diversity but still tended to center social justice issues around the experience of white women. We have the opportunity now, at the beginning of the fourth wave, to build a deeply inclusive movement.

Let's begin with a brief overview of the goals and major accomplishments of the different waves of feminism, with a focus on where each wave stood in terms of inclusivity and intersectionality.

First Wave: "Ain't I a Woman?"

The first wave of feminism in the United States spanned the nineteenth and early twentieth centuries and focused primarily on securing women's legal rights and citizenship, such as suffrage, the right to vote. The first wave covered a lot of territory in terms of women's rights. During the early nineteenth century, women and their children were considered the property of their husbands and fathers. Only white men—in most states, only white men who owned property—could vote. Throughout most of America, women were prohibited from

- Voting

- Signing legal documents

- Owning property

- Divorcing their husbands

- Attending college

- Gainful employment

The first wave of feminism originated within the abolitionist, or antislavery, movement. Originally, white women's rights activists wholeheartedly supported the end of slavery, segregation, and discrimination against black Americans, but when the Civil War ended, the women's movement experienced the first of many fractures influenced by a myopic vision of what equality meant. The fracture occurred over suffrage for black men. Although some white feminists wanted suffrage for black men, there were many who didn't. One of the most notable feminists against suffrage for black men was Susan B. Anthony (Ginzberg 2002; O'Brien 2009). Elizabeth Cady Stanton and Susan B. Anthony created the National Woman Suffrage Association (NWSA), which focused on securing the right to vote for women and excluded issues of race. In 1848, the Seneca Falls Convention, led by Elizabeth Cady Stanton and Lucretia Mott, jumpstarted the feminist movement by calling for equal treatment for women under the law, in education, and in the right to vote (Lange 2015).

After the ratification of the Fifteenth Amendment in 1870, which gave African-American men—but denied all women—the right to vote, the cause for women's suffrage gained new momentum. Still, racism was deeply embedded in the women's movement. Because they were excluded from the NWSA and other similar groups, black feminist women started their own women's rights groups, including the National Association of Colored Women (NACW). The NACW focused on issues like segregation and access to higher education in addition to black suffrage.

When the Nineteenth Amendment of the United States Constitution was passed in 1920, white women secured the right to vote, but voting was still inaccessible to women of color for many years because of discrimination and Jim Crow laws. Native American and Asian-American women were often denied citizenship, which also prevented them from voting.

But not being granted the right to vote didn't stop black feminists like Ida B. Wells from working toward equality. Wells focused on the anti-lynching movement, which was an organized effort against lynching, or the killing of a person by a mob, outside of the law. African-Americans, mostly men and boys, were targets of lynching and were often killed over false accusations of crime (such as rape and petty theft), or even killed with no justification at all (Gillis and Jacobs 2016; Brown 2003). This is a good illustration of intersectional feminism: rather than just focus on fighting for political power like their white feminist counterparts, these black women were fighting for the lives of their husbands, sons, and fathers (Nelson 2015).

The Equal Rights Amendment (ERA) was introduced in its first iteration in 1923, in this draft by Alice Paul: "Men and women shall have equal rights throughout the United States and every place subject to its jurisdiction. Congress shall have power to enforce this article by appropriate legislation." Although the phrasing has changed over time, some form of the ERA was under proposal in Congress until 1970.

In the early 1900s, a diverse group of women joined the organized labor movement. Layle Lane became the first African-American woman to serve as vice president of the American Federation of Teachers, and she worked hard for desegregation. In fact, she helped write an amicus brief supporting desegregation in the landmark 1954 Supreme Court case, Brown v. Board of Education of Topeka, in which the justices unanimously ruled that segregation in the public schools was unconstitutional. Other women in the labor movement worked toward ending sex discrimination and promoted equal pay and eight-hour workdays (Gillis and Jacobs 2016).

The controversial feminist and nurse Margaret Sanger opened the first clinic in the United States in 1916 that was focused on providing information about contraception. Under the federal Comstock Laws, enacted 1873, birth control information was deemed "obscene" and outlawed. Although Sanger was concerned about women's health and women's rights, her legacy as a feminist is complicated by her support of the eugenics movement, a racist movement that sought to sterilize women who were deemed as unfit for motherhood (Gillis and Jacobs 2016).

The racism that was steeped within first wave politics is captured powerfully by Sojourner Truth's poem, "Ain't I a Woman?" which she read at the 1851 Women's Rights Convention in Ohio. Truth's poem illustrated how the women's movement neglected the needs and experiences of women of color. Sojourner Truth pointed out how overlapping identities of race, class, and gender, weren't being considered. Truth was born a slave and later emancipated. She never learned to read or write, yet she dedicated her life to advocating for the rights of women and men.

ACTIVITY: Impact of the First Wave of Feminism

Reflect on women gaining the right to vote. How has being able to vote affected your life? Answer the questions in the space provided.

If you are able to vote, when and how did you register to vote?

_____

What did you learn from the family you grew up with about voting?

_____

_____

Are there any women in your family, from older generations, who were prevented from voting?

_____

_____

Recall the first election you voted in. What expectations did you have?

_____

_____

Do you vote in every election? Local and national? Why or why not?

_____

_____

_____

Does reading about the suffrage movement change the way you feel about voting? If so, how?

_____

_____

If you are unable to vote in the United States, write down what barriers you have to voting, and how you feel about not being able to vote.

_____

_____

_____

Second Wave: "The Personal Is Political"

The second wave of feminism emerged in the late 1960s and spanned the next decade and a half. It began in reaction to the contrived ideals of white suburban married life and the rigid gender roles found in the traditional family structure of the 1950s. Women were also frustrated by the overt sexism in the civil rights movement, especially black women who, because of their race and gender, were relegated to support and volunteer roles or were identified as the wives of civil rights leaders, such as Coretta Scott King. Women antiwar activists were also frustrated by their marginalization within the movement because of male colleagues who didn't take women's equality seriously.

Second wave feminists had a hefty agenda. They focused their work on women's liberation from discrimination and oppression, to create equal opportunities for men and women. They argued that the personal issues that women faced, like violence at home, sexual harassment at work, and unwanted pregnancies, were systemic and therefore political. This table shows the major goals and achievements of the second wave.

Second Wave Feminist Goal	Outcome
Pass the Equal Rights Amendment, giving equal rights to all citizens regardless of sex.	Did not pass. The ERA fell three states short of the required thirty-eight to amend the Constitution.
Secure protection from sexual harassment at place of employment	The federal Equal Employment Opportunity Commission was created in 1977.
Criminalize marital rape	In 1986, the federal Sexual Abuse Act made marital rape a crime on federal lands. By 1993, all fifty states had made marital rape a crime, although many states even today have marital rape exemptions or define rape in such complex ways that prosecution is difficult and rare.
Make contraception available to all women	The FDA approved the birth control pill in 1960. In 1972, the Supreme Court case Eisenstadt v. Baird made birth control available to unmarried women.
Secure equal opportunity to compete in sports	Title IX passed in 1972.
Secure right to safe and legal abortions	The landmark Supreme Court case Roe v. Wade in 1973 established this right.
End gender-based violence	Brought public attention to domestic violence as a criminal problem, not a personal, family issue. Led to the creation of rape crisis centers and battered women's shelters.
Close the pay gap	The Equal Pay Act was passed in 1963.

Second Wave Feminist Goal	Outcome
Make pregnancy discrimination unlawful in employment settings	The Pregnancy Discrimination act was passed in 1978
Offer protections for low-income women and children	The federal Supplemental Nutrition Program for Women, Infants and Children (WIC) was created in 1972.
Secure the right to serve on juries	In 1975, the Supreme Court decision in **Taylor** v. **Louisiana** prohibited women from being excluded from a jury pool.
Secure the right of women to own a credit card in their own name	The federal Equal Credit Opportunity Act passed in 1974 made it unlawful for creditors to discriminate against any applicant on the basis of sex, race, color, religion, or national origin.

A major blow to feminists during this period was the failure of the Equal Rights Amendment. The passage of the amendment was gaining momentum among the states until opponents vigorously argued against it. Ever since the introduction of the ERA by Alice Paul, opponents have thwarted passage by playing on such fears as these (Alice Paul Institute 2018)

- It would deny a women's right to be supported by her husband.

- Women would be drafted and forced into combat.

- Abortion rights would be upheld.

- Homosexual marriage would be upheld.

- Women would have to use unisex bathrooms.

With the recent resurgence of the women's movement, feminism is once again reinvigorating life into the fight for the ERA. As the deadline for ratification passed in 1982, it's possible that for the ERA to pass now, we would have to start all over again. While challenging, starting over might present an opportunity to change the language in the amendment to reflect our current understandings of the difference between gender and sex (see chapter 5).

ACTIVITY: Reflect on Feminist Goals Gained and Denied

If passed, the ERA would provide women the full protection of the Constitution and protect the legislative gains feminists have made. What does the Equal Rights Amendment mean to you?

_____

_____

_____

_____

Consider the legislation that was passed in the second wave. If you were to lose any of these rights, how would it impact your life?

_____

_____

_____

_____

SECOND WAVE ACTIVISM

Betty Friedan, author of the *Feminine Mystique*, gave voice to the unhappy suburban house-wife of the 1960s and suggested women find value and meaning in work outside the home. But, of course, low-income white women and women of color were already working outside the home and were in need of a different kind of liberation. Much like the fracture that occurred in the women's movement during the first wave, the focus on white, middle class, heterosexual women's values pushed lesbian and women of color out of the movement during the second wave. They, in turn, started their own movements focusing on issues central to their life experiences.

AIDS activism. During the 1980s, lesbians became an important part of AIDS activism. They armed themselves with education about AIDS, shared knowledge with their community about the disease, founded organizations, and developed education and prevention programs. ACT UP, an AIDS activist organization in NYC, founded by Martin Banzhaf and Alexis Danzig, fought hard for patients' rights, for accelerated drug approval for protease inhibitors, and for needle exchange programs. Lesbians were motivated to work in the organization due to the friendships they had with gay men. What was unique about ACT UP is that lesbians were treated as equals, held leadership positions within the organization, formed close friendships, and created a strong alliance against homophobia and discrimination, as they worked together to get the government to address the AIDS crisis (Wyne 2015). Lesbians and their straight allies broadened the scope of AIDS activism by lobbying for the CDC to include women and people of color in drug trials and to expand the definition of AIDS to include women.

Combahee river collective. Barbara Smith formed the black lesbian feminist collective, Combahee River Collective, in Boston, to advocate for black women's rights and seek recognition and inclusion. The collective consisted of straight, lesbian, poor black, and other women of color. In 1986 the Combahee River Collective released a statement identifying white feminism as racist and privileged and spoke out for the necessity of black women to come together as, "We realize that the only people who care enough about us to work consistently for our liberation is us." Additionally, the collective stated, "We are actively committed to struggling against racial, sexual, heterosexual, and class oppression, and see as our particular task the development of integrated analysis and practice based upon the fact that the major systems of oppression are interlocking." The collective's statement was drawing on the concept of intersectionality, as developed a decade earlier by Kimberlé Crenshaw (Webster 2017).

INTERSECTIONALITY

A critical race theorist and law professor, Kimberlé Crenshaw coined the term *intersectionality* in a 1976 employment discrimination case against General Motors to show that we can't separate a woman's experience of her gender from her race:

> Consider an analogy to traffic in an intersection, coming and going in all four directions. Discrimination, like traffic through an intersection, may flow in one direction, and it may flow in another. If an accident happens in an intersection, it can be caused by cars traveling from any number of directions and, sometimes, from all of them. Similarly, if a Black woman is harmed because she is in an intersection, her injury could result from sex discrimination or race discrimination…But it is not always easy to reconstruct an accident: Sometimes the skid marks and the injuries simply indicate that they occurred simultaneously, frustrating efforts to determine which driver caused the harm (Crenshaw 1989, 149).

The concept of intersectionality is sometimes difficult to understand because it has been used both correctly and incorrectly in different contexts. I like to think of the concept as a tool used to understand how each individual or group experiences the fight for equality. One group isn't necessarily more victimized than another (Symington 2004), and having multiple identities that experience oppression doesn't necessarily mean you experience more oppression. However, multiple layers of oppression can reinforce each other (Veenstra 2011). Additionally, some identities, like race, may be more visible or obvious than others, and other identities may be invisible, for instance, if you have a disability. Other identities may be less clear to identify, such as religion or class or if you identify as LGBTQIA. Applying an intersectional analysis to an issue helps us bring to light invisible identities and to understand the qualitatively different experience we could have from one another in the fight for equality.

Figure 1 is an example of an intersectional analysis that is centered on gender. It also demonstrates that our social identities aren't rank-ordered but are continuously changing (Collins 2000).

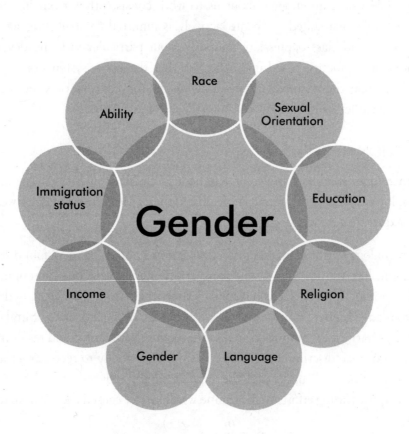

Figure 1. Gender Identity Intersectional Analysis

ACTIVITY: Visualize Your Identities

Personalize the next set of circles with some of your own identities. In the center, start with a different identity from gender and then add other identities in the smaller circles that relate to this central identity.

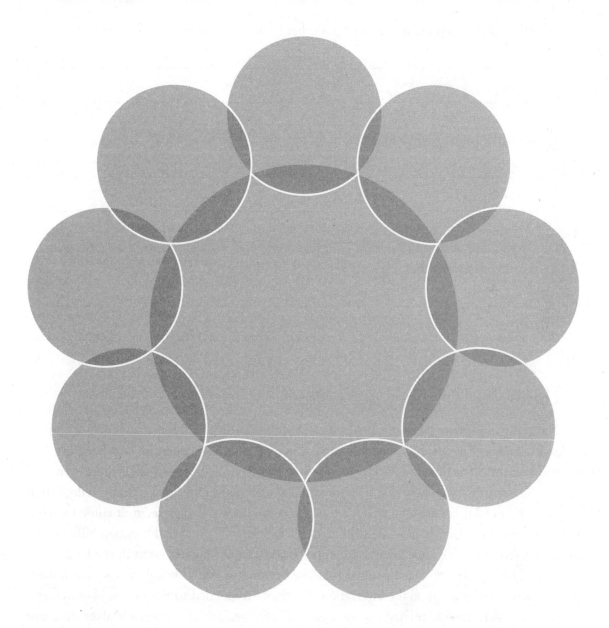

Take a moment to reflect on your visualization:

1. Which identity did you choose for the center, and why?

   _____

   _____

2. When do you tend to make identities other than gender central in your life?

   _____

   _____

3. Which of your social identities have more power? Which have less?

   _____

   _____

4. Do you ever wish your invisible identities were more visible? Do you ever wish that your invisible identities were less visible? Why or why not?

   _____

   _____

Third Wave: Changing the Culture

The third wave emerged in the 1990s, kick-started by Anita Hill's testimony in 1991, as she accused Clarence Thomas of sexually harassing her, years earlier, when he was her boss. She testified in front of the Senate Judiciary Committee, which was comprised of all white men, and it should not surprise you, now that you are familiar with patriarchy, power, and privilege, that her character quickly became the focus of the hearings. Hill was denigrated and vilified as confused and crazy. The Senate ultimately did not conclude that Thomas had harassed Hill, and he was confirmed to the Supreme Court, a lifetime position on the highest court in the land.

Anita Hill's testimony demonstrated that the personal is still political, and sexual harassment became part of a national conversation. Feminists responded to the victim blaming, and the disparaging treatment Hill had experienced, with renewed energy. Rebecca Walker, daughter of second wave black feminist writer, Alice Walker, wrote a feminist manifesto, called "Becoming the Third Wave" in Ms. *Magazine*, reacting to the ongoing discounting of women's experiences and devaluation, and reminding activists that the fight for equality is far from over (Walker 1992).

The focus in third wave feminism was less about changing legislation and more about changing the culture. The feminists of the third wave questioned and redefined gender, sex, sexuality, beauty, and language. One defining feature of third wave feminists was the emergence of *lipstick feminists* who reclaim their femininity and express their sexuality by integrating fashion and feminism. Third wave feminists also brought issues like slut shaming (stigmatizing or bullying girls and women for their sexuality), body shaming, rape culture, and sexism in the media into the national conversation. A notable distinction differentiating the third wave from other feminist movements is the influence of the growing Internet, which provided opportunities for feminists to share their ideas more broadly by blogging and publishing e-zines, laying the foundation for the current "call out culture" and constant cultural critique.

This wave of feminism brought the issues of race, class, and sexual orientation to the center, as diversity was celebrated, and intersectionality emerged as a core concept. But still white women's experience was centered over the experience of women of color. Take the common message about the gender wage gap, where women make 77 cents per every dollar that a man makes. That figure represents the pay scale for white women, and sharing this statistic, even as a means of education, puts white women at the center of discussion. In reality, women of color still make much less than white women. Additionally, third wave feminists fought to remove the glass ceiling at work. Third wave feminists focused on removing invisible barriers for women that prevented them from getting ahead in their working lives. While important, this agenda still centers the needs of white women in the movement. To include women of color, and help all women gain economic independence, third wave feminists might have focused on raising the minimum wage and expanding affordable day care options.

Here are some notable accomplishments of the third wave:

- Congress passed the Violence Against Women Act (VAWA) in 1994. VAWA was the first legislation ever to focus exclusively on ending violence against women.

- 1992 was the "Year of the Woman" because of the large number of women running for federal office and because, for the first time, four women were elected to the US Senate.

- Congress passed the Family Medical Leave Act (FMLA) in 1993 in an effort to give families more opportunities to balance family and work life, providing eligible employees up to twelve weeks of job-protected unpaid leave.

- In 1994, the military initiated a less restrictive combat position for women, opening up possibilities for more women to serve.

- Discussion of sexual harassment and rape and sexual assault became part of the cultural dialogue.

- The creation of thousands of shelters and new agencies greatly expanded women's access to rape crisis and domestic violence services.

- Feminist activism broadened to include issues that intersect with gender, such as the environment.

ACTIVITY: Third Wave Appreciation

What cultural changes that occurred during the third wave are you the most grateful for?

_____

_____

_____

_____

How do you imagine your life would be different today, if these changes hadn't happened?

_____

_____

_____

_____

Fourth Wave: Hashtag Activism

It's not exactly clear when the third wave ended and the fourth wave began. Waves are just a metaphor to understand how the goals of the feminist movement have changed and shifted over time. The fourth wave is relatively new and seems to be taking place right now and mostly online as an evolution of the call-out culture to include public cultural critiques and movements like #Metoo and #TimesUp. The #Metoo movement was initially created in 2006 by black activist Tarana Burke to call attention to the sexual violence that young women of color from low-income communities experience. The hashtag resurfaced in 2017 and gained more popularity in spreading awareness about sexual assault and harassment in the workplace.

#TIMESUP: HOW TO USE YOUR PRIVILEGE

#Timesup was created in 2018 by a group of celebrities to spread awareness of sexual harassment and assault in the workplace, particularly in Hollywood. The #Timesup organization founding committee was made up of mostly established celebrities, who hold a certain amount of power and privilege in Hollywood. Members of the Alianza Nacional de Campesinas (the National Farmworkers Alliance) reached out to the committee asking for solidarity, as female farmworkers face high levels of sexual assault and harassment. The #Timesup committee responded by publishing a letter of solidarity with farmworkers, domestic workers, service workers, and undocumented women. They also formed the #Timesup Legal Defense Fund, whose goal is to provide legal and public relations assistance to qualified individuals.

#BLACKLIVESMATTER

After the acquittal of George Zimmerman, who shot and killed Trayvon Martin, Alicia Garza wrote on her Facebook wall, "Black people. I love you. I love us. Our lives matter." Garza's friend, Patrisse Khan-Cullors, a Haiku writer, wrote, "#BlackLivesMatter" and then a movement was formed. Opal Tometi joined in to create a social media platform (Cobb 2016). Black Lives Matter centers black lives in a grassroots political and activist platform that is focused on erasing the systemic dehumanization of blacks in America and addressing systemic inequalities. Black Lives Matter is queer and trans inclusive. Although founded by three women, this movement has no central leadership or hierarchy. Black Lives Matter uses social media to bring attention to racism and violence. Attempts to discredit the movement include misinformation campaigns such as referring to #BlackLivesMatter as a terrorist organization and the release of the hashtag #AllLivesMatter. However, at its core, Black Lives Matter is a movement for peace and equality. The founders of the movement were awarded the Sydney Peace Prize in 2017.

TAKING TO THE STREETS

The fourth wave is also becoming known for protests. The *Washington Post* reported that the 2017 Women's March was most likely the largest single-day demonstration in the United States

(Chenowith and Pressman 2017). Estimates placed over one million people in Washington, DC to protest the policies and sexist behavior of newly elected president Donald Trump (Moss and Maddrell 2017; Stein, Hendrix, and Hauslohner 2017). Protesting alone doesn't cause politicians to change, but protests motivate us to get politically active and help build political movements (Madestam et al. 2013). We can see the evidence of a growing political movement as a record number of women have been running for office, and have won campaigns, since the 2017 Women's March. The protests and the number of women running for office reflect a deep-seated frustration that issues that are important to women are not being addressed (Caygle 2018).

The idea of a women's march began with a retired lawyer and educator from Hawaii, Theresa Shook, in response to the election of Donald Trump. Shook posted on Pantsuit Nation, a Facebook page in support of Hillary Clinton, that a pro-woman march was needed, and then she created a Facebook event page that attracted thousands of participants within a day. Shook originally suggested the name "Million Woman March," which was problematic because it was too similar in title to the Million Man March organized by black women in 1997. Eventually, the name was changed to the Women's March on Washington, and experienced activists were brought in to organize. After some changes in leadership, Tamika Mallory, Linda Sarsour, Carmen Perez, and Bob Bland became the organizers and faces of the Women's March.

SUCCESSES AND CHALLENGES

The 2017 Women's March on Washington was a success, with approximately five million participants worldwide. Thousands of women donned pink pussy hats as a visual symbol of solidarity. The idea of pink pussy hats came from designer Jayna Zweiman and her friend Krista Suh. According to their website, the goal was to create a visual sign of solidarity to reclaim the word "pussy" and protest against Trump's comment "Grab 'em by the pussy." The color pink was chosen as a color associated with femininity. However, the sea of pink hats, donned mostly (but not exclusively) by white heterosexual women, alienated many transgender, nonbinary, and women of color from the movement, as not all women have vulvas and not all vulvas are pink. These marginalized groups experience high rates of violence and suicide due to discrimination (James et al. 2016).

Since its inception, Women's March leaders have faced criticism from within the movement for not creating a truly inclusive movement, along with accusations of anti-Semitism and mismanagement. Clearly, creating an intersectional movement has been a challenge for feminists ever since the abolitionist movement and suffrage. Also, conflict and infighting within social justice movements are common. In social justice work, activists are highly susceptible to burnout, which can evolve into power struggles. Power struggles within activists' groups can resemble some of the conflicts the groups are working against (Chen and Gorski 2015; Plyler 2009). For instance, when a feminist group uses a top-down, hierarchal organizational structure, and members within the group are exhausted from overworking and begin competing with each other, the group can begin to feel and become patriarchal. Feminists have made and will continue to make mistakes, as this is part of being human. But we have the opportunity to learn from our mistakes, work in solidarity, and galvanize the momentum from the marches into legislative action and change. While it may be challenging to organize a movement that represents all identities, if we want change, we must make an intentional commitment to include everyone.

As we are in the midst of the fourth wave, there aren't a lot of accomplishments to list, but here are a couple of notable ones:

- All combat jobs have become open to women, without restrictions, since 2015.

- Sexual assault and sexual harassment are part of an ongoing national conversation.

- A lot of women have run for office and won!

- Feminism has been reinvigorated.

- Social justice movements, like #MeToo and #BlackLivesMatter, are linked nationally and globally, thanks to the power of technology.

ACTIVITY: Reflecting on Your Involvement

Where do you fit in as a fourth wave feminist? How do you want to fit in? Use the space provided to reflect on these questions:

Did you attend any of the 2017 Women's March events? Why or why not?

_____

_____

_____

_____

_____

_____

Did the march live up to your expectations, based on your experience of attending or reading about it?

_____

_____

_____

If you were one of the organizers, would you have done anything differently?

_____

_____

_____

_____

Reflect on the waves of feminism we covered in this chapter. What issue is important to focus on in the fourth wave? If that issue were solved, how would it impact your life? Write your thoughts down.

_____

_____

_____

FEMINIST REFLECTION

In this chapter, you explored the goals and shortcomings of the first three waves of feminism and the successes and challenges facing the fourth wave, which is happening right now. You learned how to look with an intersectional lens at social problems, which will help break the pattern of centering white women's experience in the feminist movement. You have also explored your social identities. Chapter 3 will dive into the attitudes and belief systems that help you identify as a feminist.

CHAPTER THREE

This Is What a Feminist Looks Like

"Feminism is for everybody."

—bell hooks

In 1998, I saw a film called *G.I. Jane*. Demi Moore plays a Navy SEAL recruit who is nominated by a senator as a trial candidate to see if women should be allowed to enter the Navy without restrictions. In real life, women weren't allowed to enlist as Navy SEALS until 2016. In the film, no one except perhaps the senator who nominated her expected Moore's character to pass the physically demanding training. Most men don't even make it through, so of course the assumption was that she would drop out. But she didn't. Moore's character, Jordan O'Brien, stayed committed and suffered through the intense, physically and emotionally demanding training. During one particularly grueling training, her commanding officer tells the rest of the recruits that O'Brien's presence makes them all vulnerable. Head shaved, beaten, and bloody, an exhausted and defiant O'Brien tells her commanding officer, "Suck my dick." The audience in the theater erupted with clapping and cheers. Cultural critics thought it was the best line of the movie, and critics of feminism used this scene as proof that a liberated woman is both a danger to society, for changing the nature of male-female relationships, and in danger, as men will no longer protect her (Schlafly 1997).

Was Demi Moore's character a feminist? Is "Suck my dick" a feminist mantra or, at the very least, empowering? What do you think?

Frankly, I was stunned by the audience's reaction and the commentary about the film. Up until that scene, I was impressed and inspired by the physical stamina and gender-role smashing that Moore (both the actor and her character) was committed to in the film. I was also happy that the film was directly dealing with how sexism limits roles for women. But when the audience erupted in cheers, I thought, "Wow, people are really confused about what feminism is."

Twenty years later, people are still confused about feminism.

Confusion about feminism is an outcome of a patriarchal society that defines the feminist movement through stereotypes and misinformation. If we are to believe mainstream media and critics of feminism, then *G.I. Jane* is a feminist movie because Demi Moore's character proved that she is, in fact, equal to men. But if feminism is about women being equal to men, which men should we be equal to? Not all men have power and privilege or benefit from the patriarchy (hooks 2000). Feminism isn't about women becoming equal to men. Feminism means liberation from patriarchal values and structures that are oppressive to all of us.

WHAT IS FEMINISM?

This book uses bell hooks's definition of feminism as a guiding principle of what feminism is. A black feminist theorist and social critic, hooks (who chooses not to capitalize her pen name) defines feminism as "a movement to end sexism, sexist exploitation, and oppression" (2014, 1). Her definition of feminism centers the problem clearly on sexism, and the term *movement* suggests that the solution to sexist oppression requires collective action. Although feminism focuses primarily on sexism, using an intersectional lens means that we have to account for interlocking systems of oppression, such as homophobia, anti-Semitism, white supremacy (the belief that whites are superior to other races), and classism, and how they shape experience (Hill-Collins 1990).

Misperceptions of Feminism

A movement to end sexism and oppression is beneficial for society, but to end sexism and oppression, we have to work together to dismantle patriarchal structures and other systems of oppression like racism and classism. Negative stereotypes about feminism, however, were created to dilute the message, prevent us from working together, and stall the goals of the movement. Stereotypes are an oversimplification or exaggerated truth about a group of people. For example, during the suffragist movement, which focused on securing women's right to vote, opponents used propaganda posters to spread lies about what might happen if women were able to vote, and these posters relied on negative stereotypes. They depicted unflattering images of angry women, described as "lunatics," in positions of authority over men and boys who appeared weak and powerless. These misleading and negative images of feminists have persisted for two hundred years, as society has been conditioned to believe narratives about feminists that are created by anti-feminists. Without realizing it, you may have been influenced by such stereotypes.

Anti-feminists use the radio, television, and social media, as well as other forums, to continue to spread stereotypes and misinformation about feminists. For instance, television evangelist Pat Robertson wrote the following in a fundraising letter to the Christian Coalition for the group, Stop ERA, opposing the Equal Rights Amendment in Iowa: "The feminist agenda is not about equal rights for women. It is about a socialist, antifamily, political movement that encourages women to leave their husbands, kill their children, practice witchcraft, destroy capitalism, and become lesbians" (Associated Press 1992, 16).

More recently, following the Women's March in January 2017, the media ran photos and articles about how protesters left behind a mess of garbage across the National Mall (Natelson 2017). Messy protestors were accused of being hypocrites for "not really caring about the environment" as well as demonstrating their overall "lack of class." These lies and stereotypes persisted, even though park officials disputed them and stated that the nearly five hundred thousand attendees of the March "have stacked the trash neatly as close to the [full] trash cans as they could get them" (Foley 2017). Propaganda can range from visually powerful posters distributed during suffrage to Pat Robertson's blatant lies, and can take the form of seemingly minor exaggerations such as the condition of the National Mall after the Women's March. The purpose of propaganda is to persuade an audience to believe a specific perspective, often through the use of misleading information. Propaganda is an effective tool of persuasion that influences the thoughts, attitudes, and behavior of society. Unfortunately, through propaganda, anti-feminists have led an effective campaign of spreading misinformation about feminism.

Who has influenced your perspective on feminism? Has negative propaganda played a role in your perceptions?

ACTIVITY: Identify Your Misperceptions About Feminism

Here are some common statements that contribute to a negative narrative about feminists. Check off the ones that are familiar to you:

- ☐ Feminists hate men.

- ☐ Feminists are angry all the time.

- ☐ Feminism is only for white women.

- ☐ Only women can be feminists.

☐ Feminists are ugly.

☐ Feminists like to burn bras.

☐ Feminists don't have a sense of humor.

☐ Feminists are victims.

☐ Feminists are divisive.

Consider the stereotypes that are familiar to you. Where did you first hear them? Who has influenced you? Many stereotypes of feminism come from the media or from people with power and influence who are anti-feminist yet claim to know what feminism is. Sometimes it is our friends or family who unknowingly or sometimes even knowingly spread misperceptions.

Use the chart to identify who your influencers have been, what their agenda might have been, and what you took from their message.

Influencer	Feminist or Anti-feminist Agenda	Your Take-Away Message

Write down a few thoughts on how others have influenced your ideas about feminism.

_____

_____

_____

Now that you know what anti-feminists want us to believe feminism is, and have compared it to what feminism really is, you're ready to learn how to identify sexism.

UNDERSTANDING AMBIVALENT SEXISM

Sexism is prejudice and discrimination against someone based on their gender. The definition of sexism applies to all genders. However, when considering sexism within a patriarchal society, sexism justifies and rationalizes male domination to uphold patriarchal power. The term *ambivalent sexism* describes the paradox of male and female relationships: how sexism can take hostile and benevolent forms. On one hand, there is male domination, and on the other hand, paternalistic attitudes. Patriarchal systems need sexism to justify a male-dominated society, and the gender hierarchy is maintained through both hostile and benevolent sexism (Glicke and Fiske 1996).

Hostile and Benevolent Sexism

Sexism can be an expression of hostility toward women, as in *hostile sexism*, through demeaning, derogatory, and aggressive attitudes and behaviors toward women who challenge male superiority (Glicke and Fiske 1996, 2001). Because of the aggression, hostile sexism is easy to spot. Consider the statements below that illustrate hostile sexism:

- "Women aren't as smart or as competent as men."

- "Women exaggerate their problems."

- "Women use sex to get power over men."

- "Women just want special treatment."

- "Women are manipulative."

Sexism can also be an expression of attitudes about women that may seem positive in nature but are patronizing and restrict women's roles. For example, idealizing women by considering them to be nurturers, intuitive, or natural mothers are examples of *benevolent sexism* (Glicke and Fiske 1996, 2001). Benevolent sexism offers women protection if they comply with the status quo. Benevolent sexism can sometimes come across as a compliment on the surface, but underneath the comment lie sexist beliefs that help maintain patriarchal power, by reinforcing the idea that men are more competent and should be in control. Examples of benevolent sexism include the following attitudes:

- "Women deserve men's protection."

- "Women are natural caregivers."

- "Women are delicate and sensitive."

- "Women need men to take care of them."

- "Women should be put on a pedestal."

ACTIVITY: Identify Benevolent and Hostile Sexism

Reflect on experiences that you have had with sexism. It can be a situation that you personally experienced or an experience that someone close to you has shared with you, or even something that you have heard in the news. Choose an example of benevolent sexism and an example of hostile sexism and write them down. Reflect on how these situations made you feel, either at the time you experienced the situation or how you feel now, as you are writing about the experience.

Hostile sexism example: _____

_____

Your feelings: _____

Benevolent sexism example: _____

_____

Your feelings: _____

More About Benevolent Sexism

Because benevolent sexism is typically subtler and more nuanced than hostile sexism, and seemingly well intentioned and affectionate, it can be hard to spot and easy to brush off as harmless. And to some degree, we have gotten used to and have accepted benevolent sexism as part of our lives. But this kinder, softer type of sexism is patronizing and insidious. Benevolent sexism doesn't usually trigger a coping response, because it's seemingly mild (Burgess 2013): *What's the big deal if society thinks I'm nicer or neater than I really am?* The effect being, we may not think that we need to manage or deal with benevolent sexism, which makes us more inclined to just let it go. But that is the power of benevolent sexism.

Hostile sexism motivates us to take action to stop it, but seemingly well-intentioned benevolent sexism makes us believe that we don't really have it that bad (Jost and Kay 2005). Furthermore, the idea that men take care of and protect us leads us to be less interested in participating in collective action to challenge male domination (Becker and Wright 2011).

Rewards and Punishments

Ambivalent sexism relies on a system of rewards and punishments, rewarding women who maintain the status quo and punishing women who challenge it (Glick and Fiske 2001). The term *misogyny* has been traditionally defined as hatred of women. Instead, let's think of misogyny as the enforcer of ambivalent sexism. Misogyny uses hostile sexism to keep women in their place by punishing women who challenge patriarchal norms, while also using benevolent sexism to reward women who live up to patriarchal expectations (Manne 2018).

Misogyny can enforce sexism through rewards and punishments in direct and indirect ways (Manne 2018). The following story about Amelia illustrates how we can be indirectly rewarded and punished for maintaining and challenging gendered roles in a patriarchal system:

> *Amelia is seven months pregnant and out shopping (a traditionally feminine behavior) with her two-year-old daughter in tow. While she's in the store, several strangers stop Amelia to comment on how "adorable" she looks, others touch her belly without asking, and someone lets her go ahead of them in line. People are generally warm and friendly. Amelia, however, works in this same store, and on another day, while working behind the counter, she notices that customers are not so friendly. A few people stare at her pregnant belly and then avoid eye contact with her. They don't smile at her and they keep their interactions with her short and formal. Although subtle, the message is clear: Amelia as a pregnant mom out shopping was "rewarded" with friendly behavior (oddly enough, having her belly touched without her consent) for behaving within a socially acceptable gendered way, and she was "punished" as a*

working mother for not conforming to society's roles. If Amelia were a woman of color, or queer, or disabled, she would have to deal with further discrimination.

We can also see misogyny applied in less subtle ways on an institutional level, in the sentences of incarcerated women. Women who are imprisoned for low-level nonviolent crimes are disciplined more harshly than their male counterparts. Most women who are incarcerated have mental health issues, substance abuse problems, and are trauma survivors due to histories of sexual and physical abuse. When male correction officers yell orders to a female inmate, they often respond by yelling back or shutting down and becoming silent. Most female inmates are not violent, but corrections officers respond harshly anyway, many times by sending inmates to solitary confinement over minor infractions. The officers may not consciously realize that they are enforcing a patriarchal order, but they are, by doling out harsh punishments based on their hostile views of women. Officers describe female inmates' behavior as "difficult" because they "want to communicate" and won't "take no for an answer" (Shapiro and Pupovac 2018; Reichert and Bostwick 2010). Female inmates are being punished for challenging the patriarchal structure of prisons.

In addition to doling out punishment and rewards, misogyny is a morality enforcer, which can be seen in how society splits women into categories of good or bad (Manne 2018). Good women maintain the patriarchal order, and bad women challenge it. Splitting women into categories interferes with our solidarity and ability to work together, and it creates hierarchies among women (Manne 2018).

ACTIVITY: Identifying Misogyny

Consider times that you may have heard the phrase "She's a good woman." Break down what the messaging means below. What adjectives would you use to describe a "good" woman in a patriarchal culture? What then is a "bad" woman? List those qualities too.

"Good Woman"	"Bad Woman"

The concept "slut" is a made-up social construct used to shame women for expressing their sexuality outside of patriarchal norms. This is what feminists mean by the term *slut shaming*. In reality, there's no such thing as a slut. Slut shaming is a practice of misogyny because it's used as a punishment in an attempt to reinforce acceptable behavior set by patriarchal norms.

ACTIVITY: Misogyny and Slut Shaming

Reflect on your experience with the word "slut" below:

1. When was the first time you heard this word used?

   _____

2. Who said it and why?

   _____

3. How did it make you feel?

   _____

4. Did your behavior change at all after you heard the word? Why or why not?

   _____

In a patriarchy, women, like men, are conditioned to be sexist and to maintain the patriarchal order. A predictable consequence is that we begin to believe the sexist messages and stereotypes that we are exposed to, which affects our self-esteem and also how we view and treat other women. You may have been unaware that some of the negative messages that you carry around about yourself and other women come from being conditioned to believe that women are inferior, but by now you are most likely drawing these connections. For instance, you may have low expectations about your abilities or the abilities of other women (Bearman, Korobov, and Throne 2009). There may have been times you were afraid to try something new or felt like you weren't competent enough to achieve a specific goal, or maybe you haven't felt valued by members in your family or community.

ACTIVITY: Reflecting on Internalized Sexism

Take a few moments to journal about your experiences with sexism and discrimination and any sexism that you may have internalized. Write down any insights you have gained about yourself and those experiences.

_____

_____

_____

_____

_____

The next section explores feminist attitudes and values that will help you counter the sexism that you may have internalized.

THE HOW AND WHY OF FEMINIST ATTITUDES

Feminism is an attitude, a lens through which to view the world, a collective political movement, and a way of life that is grounded in the belief that everyone is entitled to social, economic, and political equality. This section will explore how you can develop a feminist attitude and belief system. Developing a feminist perspective will help you identify the source of some of your personal struggles as a result of inequality rather than something inherently wrong with you. It is part of a personal transformation that you can make to help you deal with sexism and discrimination and free up energy, so you can take part in collective action for systemic change. We'll explore that topic later in the book. Developing a feminist attitude will require you to become aware of and decondition yourself from patriarchal messages and beliefs.

Patriarchal Vs. Feminist Schemas

Your core beliefs (or *schemas* in this book) inform and shape your attitudes. An attitude is an enduring belief that typically represents a preference for or against something. Our attitudes influence our behavior, especially if we have strong feelings about something.

Schemas represent our belief systems about the world around us and help inform our reactions to and interpretations of incoming information. Whereas attitudes express our likes or dislikes, schemas are thinking patterns that provide us with information about a person, group, or situation. Schemas are like organizational tools, or shortcuts, that we use based on our experiences. We rely on schemas to unconsciously connect present information to past information, and we do so quickly and automatically. We typically don't challenge our schemas but accept them at face value.

Schemas can be either adaptive or maladaptive, meaning that your core beliefs can be either constructive, helping you to cope with stress or upset, or not constructive, increasing your stress or upset. In the context of this book, let's consider patriarchal schemas and attitudes as maladaptive and feminist schemas and attitudes as adaptive.

Here is an example of a patriarchal schema: "Women's individual needs are no longer important once they become mothers." Here's another one: "Women are born to be mothers." Both of these schemas are maladaptive, primarily because they limit women's roles and value to motherhood and nurturing others. A patriarchal attitude based on these schemas could be *I shouldn't enjoy my job or enjoy myself when I am at social events without my children*. In this illustration, patriarchal attitudes and schemas cause stress and upset for mothers when they enjoy time away from their children, because their core beliefs, conditioned through the experience of living within a patriarchal society, tell them that they shouldn't.

Patriarchal schemas are maladaptive both on individual and societal levels. Imagine how these schemas could negatively impact you if you are an exhausted, stressed out, and sleep-deprived mother of young children, or if you have decided that motherhood isn't the right choice for you, or if you want to have children but are having fertility issues. Additionally, imagine how these schemas affect our society, in terms of policies and legislation. (Chapter 8 will look at how your personal experiences can shape your political involvement.) For now, let's begin to identify and then change, or *reframe*, these maladaptive schemas through a feminist perspective.

Here's an example of a feminist schema: "Mothers are entitled to honor their own needs." Here's another one: "Woman can lead fulfilling lives without children."

These feminist schemas are adaptive because they give you a reality check against the limiting patriarchal beliefs about women's roles. In general, the ability to identify and reframe your negative beliefs can give you a sense of greater control. We may not be able to control what happens to us in this life, but we can always control how we think about and how we interpret life events. And being able to identify your patriarchal schemas and reframe them as feminist schemas can enhance your self-esteem, as you become better able to filter out society's messages that you are inadequate (Peterson, Tantleff-Dunn, and Bedwell 2006).

Feminist Attitudes About Inequality

Feminism is a schema that influences our attitudes about inequality. Although feminism embodies a wide range of perspectives, feminists fundamentally share many similar attitudes. Here are some examples of attitudes that express feelings, thoughts, and behaviors commonly shared by feminists:

- *Gender inequality exists. I'm upset about it, and I am actively willing to challenge it.*

- *There is a connection between personal struggles and structural inequality, such as discriminatory laws and policies. I am bothered about this connection, willing to learn more about it, and am willing to challenge these inequalities for myself and others.*

- *I recognize that people may be oppressed based on their class, their ethnicity, their sexuality, their race, or their disability and understand that these different forms of oppression must all be accounted for when I challenge social, economic, and political inequality.*

ACTIVITY: Reframe a Patriarchal Schema

Remember a time that you heard a sexist message. Write it down below, and then consider the message from a feminist perspective. Cross out the sexist message and rewrite it from a feminist perspective. For example, prior to getting my undergraduate education, I was once told by an elder relative, "It's a waste of money for women to get an education." Fortunately, I already identified as a feminist and went on to earn a doctoral degree anyway. In my mind, I identified the comment as sexist, and reframed the message to be *I am entitled to get the education that I want, and your sexism isn't going to stop me.*

Sexist schema: _____

_____

Feminist reframe: _____

_____

Developing your own feminist schema will help you decondition yourself from patriarchal values, learn to interpret and respond to incoming information quickly, and reject sexist messages.

ATTITUDES AND ATTRIBUTION THEORY

Your attitudes and feminist schema will to some degree determine how you interpret or explain the cause of behavior or events. According to attribution theory, typically when looking at our own lives, we attribute our behavior to situational events, and when looking at others' behavior, we attribute their behavior to something internal (Fiske and Taylor 1991). For example, when you get angry and lose your temper, you're likely to blame your behavior on an outside event like stress from work. But when you see someone else lose their temper, you are more likely to assume it's because of their temperament. Generally, this means that we tend to overemphasize the personal characteristics of others and neglect to consider the context or situational factors that may be affecting their behavior. Except when it comes to discrimination.

ATTRIBUTIONS AND DISCRIMINATION

When experiencing discrimination, women are more likely to be reluctant to identify a behavior as discriminatory, particularly if the source of the discrimination is another person, and especially if that person might experience a negative consequence from having their sexist behavior called out (Sechrist and Delmar 2009).

Consider this example. You are on a break at work, chatting about your weekend casually with your coworkers. Your male colleagues joke that you're probably still single because of your "attitude." You're not sure what attitude they are referring to, and because they were laughing, you aren't sure if they are serious or not. You may walk away feeling uncomfortable and confused.

How will you interpret this situation? From a feminist perspective, consider the following:

1. What role did your gender play in this scenario? For example, would your male coworkers make the same kind of comment to each other?

2. What if you are a person of color? If so, did the reference to your "attitude" make you wonder if they were making a racialized remark based on stereotypes of black women being angry or Latinas' "spiciness"?

3. What might the outcome be for you and for your colleagues if you state simply, "That comment sounds sexist"?

You may never fully know the answer to these questions, but how you interpret this situation can affect how your feel about yourself. If your automatic reaction is to walk away feeling self-conscious about how others perceive you, and you tend to blame yourself for this interaction, you're likely to feel bad about yourself and possibly embarrassed or even ashamed for interacting casually with your coworkers.

IT'S NOT YOU, IT'S THE PATRIARCHY

Now take the same scenario and imagine responding to it as a feminist. What if your automatic reaction were to see your male coworker's comments as inappropriate, sexist, and perhaps racist, rather than respond as if there were something inherently wrong with you. You would likely attribute the situation to sexism and discrimination, and you would be more likely to walk away still feeling good about yourself (Major, Quinton, and Schmader 2003).

Over time, as you develop your feminist perspective, learning how to react differently in the moment will come more easily. It may also help to identify a feminist role model who can inspire you with their attitudes and behaviors. To increase the likelihood that this next exercise will make you feel good about yourself and raise your self-esteem, the person you choose should identify as the same gender as you and be like you in some way (Wohlford, Lochman and Barry 2004).

ACTIVITY: Identify a Feminist Role Model

Do some research to identify someone who can be a feminist role model for you, based on their attitudes and behaviors.

Who is your role model? _____

What do you admire about this person? _____

_____

_____

How does your role model express their feminism? _____

_____

_____

Brittney Cooper (2018) wrote about the collective superpowers of black women's eloquent rage to fuel their fight against inequality. Perhaps what you and your role model have in common is a certain *feminist superpower*. Your superpower is a special set of skills that you have and can bring to the feminist movement to support change. There's no skill too large or small! List your superpower below.

_____

_____

_____

FEMINIST REFLECTION

In this chapter, you explored what feminism is, along with the misperceptions of feminism and why they exist. You looked at how sexism is used to justify male domination and how misogyny enforces compliance within the patriarchal system. Lastly, we worked on how you can develop your own feminist identity and began to discuss why it is beneficial to you. The next chapter will explore more deeply the effects that sexism has on the mental health of women.

CHAPTER FOUR

Sexism, Discrimination, and Mental Health

"Women have been trained to think that we are overreacting or that we're being too sensitive or unreasonable."

—Tracee Ellis Ross

In *Everyday Sexism*, Laura Bates (2016) recounts being groped, followed off a bus, yelled at from a car, and having her hand grabbed and held by a man in a café—all in the span of one week. Bates refers to these events as her tipping point, not because these experiences were unique but because they were all too familiar. Wondering why she'd always felt that she needed to put up with normalized harassment and sexism, Bates began asking all of the women she knew whether they had encountered similar experiences, and, of course, they had.

However, in her conversations with these women, the feedback she was largely getting was that sexism is dead, women are "mostly equal" anyway and therefore don't have reason to complain, and that what women really need to do is lighten up. To combat the invisibility of normalized, everyday sexism, in 2012, Bates began the Everyday Sexism Project, a website dedicated to cataloguing the stories of sexism that women experience daily. By 2015, Everyday Sexism had received over a hundred thousand submissions from girls as young as eight and from women of all ages around the world. The stories that have been submitted range from daily instances of sexist comments to stories of violence including abuse and rape (Bates 2016).

The Everyday Sexism Project documents what Bates calls "the drip-drip-drip of sexism" that women experience against a backdrop of denial, where society tells us that what we are experiencing isn't actually happening or that our experiences aren't a big deal and we should just laugh it off. This is a form of gaslighting, meaning that it makes us question our own experience and reality, so it's no wonder that sexism and discrimination are major vulnerability factors for stress and physical and mental illness.

ACTIVITY: Your Tipping Point

Reflecting on Bates's experience, consider what your own tipping point is (or was). When did your experience with sexism and discrimination become significant enough to motivate you to change or challenge the status quo? Write about your tipping point below:

_____

_____

_____

_____

_____

_____

_____

This chapter will explore the effects of sexism by looking at a progression of gendered experiences ranging from the chronic stress that results from discrimination and the everyday accumulation of sexist comments and insults to the effects of gender-based violence. On the surface, the connection between sexist comments, discrimination, and gender-based violence may not be obvious, but these experiences are connected because lower-level sexism creates a foundation of mistreatment for women and girls, which supports a culture of violence, and these are the experiences most likely to affect your mental health. As you read on, you may find that certain experiences of discrimination resonate with you and others don't. For the experiences that don't resonate with you, use the information and exercises as a way to understand these issues more deeply and learn how to be an effective ally for others.

DON'T CALL US CRAZY

A common trope of anti-feminists and sexists is to call women crazy or hysterical when we call out sexism. Our stories and experiences should be enough to convince ourselves and others of the pervasiveness of sexism and its effects on our lives. For further validation, sexism and its effects have been documented through extensive research.

Sexism is damaging to women's physical and mental health. Women and girls experience discrimination ranging from mundane, everyday events, like street harassment, slut shaming, and the lack of equitable division of labor in heterosexual marriages, to extreme events including threats of and actual gender-based violence (Bearman, Korobov, and Thorne 2009; Swim et al. 2001). Sexism is a stressor that leads to lowered confidence and self-esteem and is linked to psychological distress (Zucker and Landry 2007). Women are diagnosed at higher rates with depression, anxiety disorders, somatic complaints (such as chronic pain), post-traumatic stress disorder (PTSD), and eating disorders (Astbury 2001; McLean et al. 2011). And doctors often dismiss or ignore women's concerns about pain (Hoffmann and Tarzian 2001). Women outnumber men with diagnosed mental health disorders in part because women are more likely to seek treatment than men and in part because of gender stereotyping in diagnosis (Ali, Caplan, and Fagnant 2010).

Sexism and oppression are both a cause and an effect of stress. For instance, women's lower status in society creates gender-based risk factors for psychiatric disorders and psychological distress, which in turn increases the likelihood of oppression and inequality. Below are risk factors for psychiatric disorders and psychological distress that are a result of gender inequality (Astbury 2001):

- Women make up the bulk of the world's poor.

- Women earn less than men, which may lead to the chronic stress of insecure housing, reduced social support, and dependence on others.

- Low social status is a predictor of depression.

- Violence against women is a worldwide epidemic.

Other damaging aspects of gender-based discrimination include internalizing messages of blame and lowered self-worth and self-confidence from living in a culture that devalues you.

SEXISM IS STRESSFUL

Stress is a state of mind that involves both the body and the brain in reaction to a perceived threat or challenge to your ability to meet your real or perceived needs (McEwen 2012; Greenberg, Carr, and Summers 2002). A stressor is a threatening event that causes a stress response.

Women experience more stress than men, a significant factor in our high rates of anxiety, heart disease, and insomnia (Wong 2018). Below are some examples of everyday gender-based stressors that contribute to women's high stress levels (Berg 2006).

- Being treated unfairly because of your gender

- Being the recipient of unwanted sexual advances

- Being primarily responsible for child care in addition to employment

- Being the primary caregiver for a family member

- Being responsible for doing the work of emotional labor or caretaking within your relationship(s) and family

- Experiencing gender-based violence

- Working in a male-dominated field

ACTIVITY: Identify Your Gender-Based Stressors

Have you experienced anything in the preceding list of everyday gender-based stressors? Reflect on any experiences that come to mind.

_____

_____

_____

_____

_____

List any other gender-based stressors that you have experienced that were not in the preceding list:

_____

_____

_____

Which gender-based stressors have you experienced most often?

_____

_____

_____

Which gender-based stressors have had the most impact on you?

_____

_____

_____

If you identify with a marginalized group, how does that identity magnify your experience of gender-based stress?

_____

_____

_____

_____

Fight, Flight, or Freeze

How we react to a stressor is based on our individual biology, our psychology, our lifestyle, and our lived experiences (McEwen 2012; Jackson 2013). But what we all have in common is a built-in, automatic stress response system, called the *autonomic nervous system*, which is the body's way of adapting to and responding to stress.

Your autonomic nervous system is part of your body's stress response system, and it becomes engaged when you are exposed to a stressor. There are two branches of the autonomic nervous system, the *sympathetic* and the *parasympathetic* nervous system. Through the release of stress hormones, the sympathetic nervous system activates your fight-or-flight system, to fight back or flee. The parasympathetic nervous system usually operates when your body is at rest, preparing the body to relax and conserve energy. However, the experience of terror or extreme fear can activate the sympathetic and parasympathetic system simultaneously, which triggers a freeze reaction. We may freeze in response to a traumatic event.

Without training (such as that received in martial arts or the military), we can't control how our body responds to a stressor. And sometimes even with training we can't control how our body will react to stress. Often our body will take over and respond in the way that will most likely maintain our safety.

ACTIVITY: Your Stress Response

Looking at the gender-based stressors you identified in the previous exercise, was your response in each case to fight, fly, or freeze? This chart lists the symptoms of each type of response. Check off the responses that resonate the most with you. Then write down which gender-based stressors have triggered your fight, flight, or freeze response.

Fight	Flight	Freeze
Feelings of anger or rage	Desire to run or hide	Feeling unable to move
Desire to hit or kick	Desire to escape	Holding your breath
Yelling	Feeling fidgety	Isolating yourself
Breathing faster or deeper	Surrendering	Dissociating (zoning out, going numb, or retreating into fantasy)
Crying	Feeling anxiety	
Becoming confrontational		Feeling helpless
Feeling defensive		

Fight	Flight	Freeze
Stressor:	Stressor:	Stressor:

Take a moment to reflect on the connections you have made so far between your stressors and your fight, flight, or freeze response. What insights have you gained from reflecting on how sexism affects you?

_____

_____

_____

_____

The Role of Resiliency

Although the body is prepared to adapt to stressors in the short term, chronic long-term exposure to stress can leave us vulnerable to disease. Sexism, discrimination, and oppression are examples of chronic long-term stress, which explains why sexism can affect women's mental and physical health. Discrimination is the experience of being treated differently based on your social identity (Kreiger 2005), and some forms of discrimination may have more negative effects than generic stress, for example, if tied to the parts of you that are unchangeable, like your race. Discrimination is personal and demeaning (Zucker and Landry 2007; Landrine and Klonoff 1996), which can make you feel even more distressed. *Resiliency* is the ability to bounce back after adversity and stress. Recognizing and acknowledging stress from discrimination, and how it affects you, will help you manage your stress better. Chapter 9 will look more deeply at the role of self-care, and how taking care of yourself, your needs, and feelings will improve your resiliency, which in itself is an act of resistance.

SEXIST MICROAGGRESSIONS

Most sexism and discrimination is felt in lower level and subtle ways in the form of *microaggressions*. These are everyday insults or subtle communications of prejudice, hostility, and discrimination that may or may not be intentional. An occasional insult here or there isn't enough to cause chronic stress, but microaggressions accumulate and can affect your mental health and quality of life. Microaggressions also maintain a social group's marginalization (Sue et al. 2007). African-Americans and other racial minorities experience more microaggressions than whites, often on a daily basis (Andrade 2013). The experience of daily, personal, sexist interactions may result in trauma symptoms, leave women vulnerable for retraumatization, and potentially increase the likelihood of a diagnosis of PTSD (Berg 2006; Pinquart and Sörensen 2006).

The concept of microaggressions was originally intended to describe the "subtle and stunning" racist messages that people of color experience incessantly everyday (Pierce 1970, 266), although any marginalized group can experience microaggression and its effects (Sue 2010).

ACTIVITY: Your Experience with Microaggressions

Check off any these microaggressions that you have experienced.

- ☐ Being called "bossy," "bitchy," or "shrill"
- ☐ Told you are "overreacting," "crazy," or "too sensitive"
- ☐ When you are upset, being asked if you are on your period
- ☐ Getting unsolicited comments on your choice of clothing
- ☐ Receiving comments on your body size

- [ ] Being told that you are "too old" to date, wear certain clothes, or work

- [ ] Being told "You throw or run like a girl"

- [ ] Hearing a comment like "Wow, you're strong for a woman!"

- [ ] Told you would look pretty if you "smiled more"

List any other microaggresssions that you would add from your experience:

_____

_____

_____

Who are you most likely to hear microaggressions from and in what context (such as your boss when you ask for time off or from your partner when you express your feelings)?

_____

_____

_____

_____

_____

How do you feel when you are the recipient of a microaggression?

_____

_____

_____

Note that subtle discrimination and sexism is real and common, but not everyone experiences stress or upset from microaggressions. Microaggressions are subjective and ambiguous. More research is needed to clarify the definition of microaggressions and to understand better who is more affected by subtle discrimination and why (Lilienfeld 2017).

Handling Microaggressions in the Moment

One of the reasons that microaggressions can be so frustrating is that we don't always know how to respond or even if we should. And the fight-or-flight response (to be confrontational or to pretend it didn't happen) can make the situation worse and increase your stress.

However, you can use direct communication in the moment or after experiencing a microaggression to proactively defend yourself against microaggressions, invisibility, and unequal power (Irey 2013). Using direct communication can also create meaningful dialogue about sexism. This section will look at three different kinds of direct communication that work well in these situations. Note that these strategies of everyday resistance may be experienced as confrontational, which may or may not be the right response for you based on the situation. For example, a direct confrontation may not be the best choice in some work contexts or in any situation where the consequence could be severe (loss of employment, further discrimination, violence). Any of these strategies can be adapted and used to advocate for yourself or to be an ally for someone else.

OPEN THE FRONT DOOR TO COMMUNICATION

Open the front door (OTFD) to communication addresses microaggressions directly (Cheung, Ganote, and Souza 2016) using the following steps:

Observe: Observe what just happened, based on facts, without an interpretation.

Think: Describe what you think or what others may think about the interaction.

Feel: Express your feelings using an *I-message*. For example, "I feel…when you say or do this."

Desire: Request your desired outcome.

Let's look at an example of a microaggression where you could apply this kind of direct communication.

Imagine you are a middle-aged lesbian woman who is multiracial. You appreciate fashion, and are always dressed impeccably, and you usually receive many compliments on your sense of style.

One day you're at work and during casual conversation, a colleague asks you about your husband. You reply, "I don't have a husband, actually. I'm a lesbian."

Your colleague replies with surprise, "But you don't look like a lesbian."

This is a classic and common microaggression about lesbian women, the underlying assumption being that lesbians should look a certain way.

Here's how you would apply OTFD in this situation:

Observe: "I noticed that you made a stereotypical statement about lesbians. I've heard you make statements like this before."

Think: "It's not unusual for people unfamiliar with LGBTQIA folk to rely on stereotypes for information."

Feel: "I feel uncomfortable and frustrated hearing stereotypes about me and my social identity that aren't true."

Desire: "I'd like to understand more about why you said you are surprised."

ACTIVITY: Try Out OTFD

Think about a microaggression that was directed at you. Describe the microaggression.

_____

_____

_____

_____

_____

_____

How would you respond using the OTFD model?

Observe: _____

Think: _____

Feel: _____

Desire: _____

Create Cognitive Dissonance

Another form of direct communication is to create *cognitive dissonance* in the speaker. Cognitive dissonance refers to the discomfort caused by inconsistent attitudes and behavior. People are often motivated to change either their attitude or their behavior when they feel this discomfort (Gruber 2003). You can create cognitive dissonance during a conversation with this communication template: "I'm surprised to hear you say something [racist/homophobic/sexist] as I've always thought you were [open-minded/an ally/supportive]."

ACTIVITY: Try Out Cognitive Dissonance

Using one of the microaggressions you have experienced, try out how you might create cognitive dissonance in the speaker. Write down what you might say.

_____

_____

_____

_____

Ask Clarifying Questions

A third method of direct communication is to ask for clarification. For example, you respond to a microaggression by asking "Can you explain what you mean by that?" or "Where did you get that idea?"

Tip: Keeping your voice even is key to making this a lower-level confrontational strategy.

ACTIVITY: Try Out Clarifying Questions

Using another microaggression that you have experienced, try out a clarifying question. What might you ask?

Microaggression: _____

Clarifying question: _____

NONCONFRONTATIONAL MICRORESISTANCE

In instances when a direct confrontation is not in your best interest, try using some of the strategies below, either individually or in collaboration with others. The strategies below have been used as active resistance and are focused more on addressing structural inequalities than on changing an individual's behavior (Irey 2013).

- Seeking out mentors and role models within and outside of work

- Becoming a mentor or role model

- Social networking with an affinity group

- Consciously challenging stereotypes about your gender, race, sexual orientation, and social class

- Taking a leadership role in your community, to be less invisible

- Demonstrating a different leadership model, one that is empowering, collaborative, and resists structural oppression

GENDER-BASED VIOLENCE

In this section, I will be using the expressions "gender-based violence" and "violence against women" somewhat interchangeably. In general, the term gender-based violence refers to violence against women, but it also can include violence that is directed toward someone's gender or gender expression, for instance, people who are transgender or nonbinary. In cases where research and statistics on violence are focused on violence against women, specifically, I use the expression "violence against women." Additionally, in this section, I am focused on relational and sexual violence. Chapter 6 will explore body oppression, which includes violence that is directed toward people's intersecting identities.

Chronic stress from everyday sexism, inequality, microaggressions, and stereotypes may not on the surface seem connected to gender-based violence, but they are in the sense that sexist jokes, insults, and behavior provide the foundation that supports gender-based violence. In fact, the way to reduce gender-based violence is to promote gender equality (World Health Organization 2009). All forms of sexism are expressions of inequality, and lower-level sexism is the base from which violence grows. Violence and the threat of violence impact girls' and women's lives dramatically. Violence against women is also a major contributing factor for the high rates of PTSD and depression among girls and women. Young women, women of color, indigenous women, undocumented women, poor women, and trans women are all particularly vulnerable to violence and are victimized at disproportionally high rates. To understand why violence affects women's mental health, it's important to understand how and to what degree violence, and the threat of violence, along with societal blame and self-blame, affect women's lives and recovery.

Violence against women is so prevalent worldwide that it has been accepted as an inevitable fact in women's lives (Susmitha 2016). Violence against women affects every aspect of women's lives, to the degree that it is a human rights violation, and should be regarded as such (Kaur and Garg 2008). But if you have experienced violence or the threat of violence in your life, chances are that you have minimized or denied it, blamed yourself, felt compassion for the abuser, tried to change your behavior to keep yourself safe, felt weak, experienced symptoms of PTSD, and had to put most of your energy and efforts into keeping your life together, protecting your children if necessary, and just generally surviving.

Rape and Sexual Assault

According to the National Intimate Partner and Sexual Violence Survey, one in three women experience sexual violence at some point in their lives (Smith et al. 2017), and one in five women reports being raped during their lifetime (Breiding, Chen, and Black 2014). The umbrella term "sexual assault" includes rape, attempted rape, sexual coercion, unwanted sexual contact like touching or groping, and unwanted sexual experiences like harassment and stalking (Smith et al. 2017). Sexual assault is one of the most traumatic experiences you can have, which is why it is strongly associated with PTSD (Kessler et al. 2005). Sexual assault can cause symptoms of depression, somatic symptoms, alcohol abuse, and disordered eating (Yuan, Koss, and Stone 2006).

IMPACT OF RAPE CULTURE AND RAPE MYTHS

The inevitability of most women to experience some kind of sexual assault illustrates how normalized sexual violence is in our culture. In a rape culture, everyday sexism and mistreatment of women, sexual violence is normalized, trivialized, and victims are blamed.

Here are some examples of how rape and sexual assault are normalized and trivialized in our culture.

- Jokes about sexual assault, stalking, or sexual harassment

- Using expressions like "Boys will be boys" to minimize or rationalize sexist and/or violent behavior

- Blaming rape or sexual assault on what women wear

- Using vague language like "nonconsensual touching" or "nonconsensual intercourse" instead of naming what it is: sexual assault or rape

- Instituting dress code policies in schools so that girls don't distract boys

- Assuming women are lying or exaggerating about their experience with sexual violence

- Rape-validating lyrics in songs (such as "You know you want it")

- Gratuitous rape scenes in movies and television

- Hypersexualization of girls and women in movies, television, and the media

- Slut shaming

- Rape prevention programs that are focused on women's choices (such as carrying mace or other weapons or not traveling alone at night) rather than on men changing their behavior

ACTIVITY: Recognizing Rape Culture

What examples of rape culture have you witnessed or experienced? Reflect on what messages you have internalized about women and sexual assault or rape. How have these messages impacted you?

_____

_____

_____

_____

_____

_____

_____

Victim blaming and the perpetuation of rape myths contribute to the development of PTSD in sexual assault victims (Chivers-Wilson 2006). Rape myths are widespread beliefs and attitudes about rape that rationalize sexual violence, reduce empathy for the victim, and shift the blame for sexual assault away from the perpetrator to the victim. An example of a rape myth is "No really means yes" or "Only strangers are rapists." Hearing rape myths can retraumatize survivors and prevent reporting (Edwards et al. 2011). A belief in rape myths is also common in men who commit sexual assault (Desai, Edwards, and Gidycz 2008). Rape myths are an outgrowth of a patriarchal system.

Rape myths are so pervasive and automatic that when we hear stories of sexual assault, we are conditioned to find ways to blame the victim. Consider Alix's story:

Alix was hanging out with friends after work one night at a local bar. Alix had a couple of drinks and was having fun. She decided to invite everyone back to her apartment to continue the party. At some point during the evening, she began kissing the friend of a coworker. Soon they were in Alix's bedroom, and they fooled around some more. Alix took her top and pants off but left on her bra and underwear. Alix said no when asked if she would take her underwear off. Because of the alcohol, both fell asleep. Alix woke up in the middle of the night to realize that she was being raped. Groggy and still slightly intoxicated, Alix froze with fear and couldn't move or speak. Afterward, Alix lay in bed awake and unsure of what to do or say. The acquaintance who had raped her fell back asleep.

ACTIVITY: Identifying Rape Myths

Reread Alix's story, and check off which rape myths come to mind:

☐ No really means yes.

☐ Saying yes to getting undressed implies consent for everything.

☐ Alix was "asking for it" by taking her clothes off.

☐ Only strangers are rapists.

☐ It's only rape if the victim physically fights or resists.

☐ If it's a real rape, the victim will be extremely upset or even hysterical afterward.

☐ You can't be raped if you're under the influence of alcohol.

☐ It's the woman's fault for drinking too much.

☐ Only men can be rapists (notice in Alix's story that the gender of the perpetrator was not revealed).

☐ It's only rape if a weapon was used.

It's possible to be aware that rape isn't the victim's fault and yet still find ways to blame the victim for being raped. This is because we have been conditioned to blame or disbelieve rape victims. Reflect on the messages that you have received or internalized from living in a patriarchal society that normalizes violence against women. How have those messages impacted you and your reactions to sexual assault and rape?

_____

_____

_____

_____

_____

TONIC IMMOBILITY AND THE FREEZE RESPONSE

Alix's story illustrates a common way sexual assault survivor respond during an attack or when exposed to an extreme threat. They respond much like many animals do, which is to freeze and become immobile. This phenomenon is referred to as *tonic immobility*, which is an adaptive defense mechanism that temporarily prevents you from resisting or physically fighting back. Earlier in the chapter, I referred to this freeze response, which occurs when your sympathetic and parasympathetic nervous system are engaged simultaneously. During tonic immobility, it's also common to feel a sense of calm, because your body produces an analgesic effect (Möller, Söndergaard, and Helström 2017).

After an assault, survivors may be confused and feel ashamed by what they perceive as their lack of resistance, and this self-blame increases their vulnerability to being diagnosed with PTSD. In my therapy practice, most of the sexual assault victims I have worked with over the years have experienced tonic mobility during and after the sexual assault, which resulted in deep feelings of shame and self-blame. Tonic immobility is the body's way of defending itself during a situation that you can't escape. Unfortunately, the body's freeze response plays right into the hands of a culture that wants to blame rape victims, particularly those who don't "fight back" in a way that society understands or accepts.

LIVING UNDER THE THREAT OF VIOLENCE

In general, women are more afraid of yet less likely to be a victim of crime than men, with the exception of intimate partner violence and sexual assault. Women live under the shadow of sexual assault, a theory that describes women's general fear of crime being due to the belief that any crime can lead to a sexual assault (Fisher and Sloane 2003; Özascilar 2013). Living with the constant threat of sexual assault is a chronic stressor, which leads women to become hypervigilant. To reduce the risk of sexual assault, women often organize their lives in some way to avoid being the victim of violence. Although the rates of victimization of sexual assault and intimate partner violence are high, and women's fear is realistic, women are also socialized to believe that the risk of sexual assault is constant, especially at night (Lane and Meeker 2003). Many strategies that women use to stay safe from sexual assault are inherently victim blaming, as they place the burden on women to prevent rape, while maintaining a rape culture that normalizes violence against women as an inevitable fact of life (Buchwald, Fletcher, and Roth 1993). Women's constant fear of violence contributes to the endorsement of benevolent sexism, particularly the belief that women need to be protected (Phelan, Sanchez, and Broccoli 2010).

The threat of rape is so prevalent in women's lives that we engage in strategies every day to minimize the chance that we will be assaulted. The strategies that we use are reinforced by exposure to "rape prevention tips" that are directed at woman to reduce the likelihood of being sexual assaulted (Bedera and Nordmeyer 2015). Here are some strategies many women engage in to avoid sexual assault:

- Avoiding certain places, especially at night

- Avoiding going out alone

- Taking a self-defense class

- Alter your clothing choices

- Avoid public transportation

- Double- or triple-checking that the door is locked (car door, front door)

- Carrying a weapon (mace, a pocket knife, or gun)

ACTIVITY: Common Ways Women Protect Themselves from Sexual Assault

Consider how the threat of sexual violence has impacted your quality of life and your level of stress.

In what ways do you protect yourself from sexual assault and other types of violence? Do you use any of the common strategies in the preceding list? Do you have other strategies?

_____

_____

_____

Are there activities that you avoid to reduce your risk of sexual assault?

_____

In what ways does making decisions based on your safety affect your level of stress and quality of life?

_____

_____

_____

What messages can you take from this section on rape and sexual assault that will help you decondition from patriarchal victim-blaming messages?

_____

_____

_____

_____

Intimate Partner Violence

When you hear the term *intimate partner violence*, what image comes to mind? Do you think of physical abuse? Intimate partner violence (IPV) includes psychological abuse, intimidation and coercive control, stalking, rape and sexual assault and physical assault (Breiding, Chen, and Black 2014). Violence in our intimate relationships is the most common type of violence that women experience (Tjaden and Thoennes 2000). Intimate partner violence (IPV) is a complex social issue that is caused by the influences of many well-documented factors, including gender inequality, social norms and mores, patriarchal family structures, politics and policies, the media, structural supports such as families and religious institutes, schemas and attitudes about violence and gender roles, violence in the family of origin, psychiatric illness, lack of emotion regulation skills by the perpetrator, poverty and stress, and social learning (Breiding, Chen, and Black 2014; Lohman et al. 2013; Namy et al. 2017; Susmitha 2016). Both women and men can be victims of IPV, and at nearly similar rates, but women are more likely to be physically harmed (Tjaden and Thoennes 2000). They are also more likely to experience extreme forms of physical violence, such as being kicked, choked, suffocated, beaten, or burned; IPV can occur among couples in every race, class, and sexual orientation (Breiding, Chen, and Black 2014). Women and girls are at risk of experiencing violence in their relationships around the world. The World Health Organization (2013) estimates that one in three women will experience intimate partner violence in their lifetime.

The potential effects on women's mental health and quality of life range in severity, depending upon whether or not the abuse was a single incident or is chronic and lasting over a lifetime. Plus, if you have experienced childhood abuse, or have a history of rape or sexual assault, the risk of physical and mental health conditions is significantly higher. Living with violence affects women's emotional and physical health and undermines their economic and social well-being (Susmitha 2016).

Women who have experienced IPV are more likely to experience these conditions (Breiding, Chen, and Black 2014; Susmitha 2016):

- Anxiety

- PTSD

- Physical injury

- Low self-esteem

- Suicide attempts

- Gastrointestinal disorders, such as irritable bowel disorder

- STIs

- Gynecological or pregnancy complications and menstrual issues

- Binge-drinking

- Smoking

- Risky behaviors that increase the likelihood of HIV

- Missing work or school

- Headaches

- Chronic pain

- Difficulty sleeping

- Asthma

- Diabetes

- Overall poor health

- Disrupted family life

- Poverty

- Interrupted educational and career paths

- Belief that men are superior to women

- Distrust of men

Share Your Story

Many victims of IPV don't tell their stories because of shame and self-blame as well as the fear that the person you disclose to will also shame you, not believe you, invalidate your experience, or blame you for what happened (Sylaska and Edwards 2014). But if you are a victim of any gender-based violence, disclosing your experience to supportive friends or family can be a positive and helpful way to take control of your recovery and reduce negative effects on your health from keeping your story a secret. Sharing your story is also a powerful way to affect people and their perceptions of violence against women. It's not necessary as a feminist to publicly disclose your experience with violence. However, if you are even considering publicly disclosing your experience in the future, it's a good idea to practice talking about your experience now, by confiding in supportive people with whom you feel safe.

Consider who in your life would be a safe and supportive person to tell? Do you have a feminist ally to talk to? Who is likely to not judge you and to understand? If you don't feel safe sharing your story with friends or family, consider joining a group with other survivors.

Before you share your story, be clear about what you need from the person who is listening. Your initial conversation could go like this: "I'd like to talk to you about something that is very personal to me, and I'm not used to talking about it. What I need from you is to listen and not judge."

And remember, you are in charge of what you tell and what you don't tell. You don't have to share all the details. You are in control of your story.

FEMINIST REFLECTION

In this chapter, you've explored how sexism and inequality can be damaging to your mental health, self-esteem, and quality of life. You now understand the role that everyday sexism and discrimination plays in some of your actual—and feared—life experiences and have identified some of your own gender-based stressors. You've also explored how gender-based violence affects you. In part 2, you will learn how to actively identify and challenge inequality. Chapter 5 focuses on the social construction of gender and how perceiving gender as binary is a tool of the patriarchy.

PART 2

GETTING WOKE AND STAYING WOKE

CHAPTER FIVE

The Future Is a Spectrum

"How about we stop separating the children into opposing teams from day dot? How about we give them seven to ten years to consider themselves on the same side?"

—Hannah Gadsby

Alex races into the classroom, out of breath from running very late, and quickly grabs a seat near the door. Distracted by this, you stop taking notes and watch as Alex sits down. Alex is tall with lean muscles and dark curly hair. Releasing a sigh, Alex takes out a pen, opens a notebook, and right away raises a hand to ask a question.

What image of Alex's gender comes to mind? Did you visualize a male or a female? Or perhaps someone who identifies as queer, or not necessarily male or female? How did you make this determination? Are there any key words or impressions that helped you form an image of Alex that was decidedly one gender and not the other?

Gender is so deeply entrenched in our collective unconscious that reading the description of Alex, which does not include Alex's gender, you likely made an automatic assumption about Alex's gender without even being aware of it. Most readers would choose male or female. Our automatic assumptions about gender typically reflect societal expectations about men and women.

In this chapter, we will explore the ways in which culture leads us to internalize stereotypes about gender. The goal is to understand how our culture reinforces men and women to exist in separate categories, and how this separation is a tool of the patriarchy, because a gender binary supports a social hierarchy. In terms of gender, your part in dismantling the patriarchy is to allow yourself the flexibility to see how gender roles can limit you in your life, and to find the places where you are willing to step out of your comfort zone and challenge the patriarchal narrative that men and women are separate genders on opposing teams. To do so will give you the freedom to be yourself without preconceived notions of who you should be.

MYTHS ABOUT MEN AND WOMEN

There are differences between men and women, but we are more alike than not. Men and women are alike in most characteristics, such as our personality and cognitive abilities (APA 2005). The major organs in our bodies, such as the brain, kidneys, and heart, are all unisex organs (Eliot 2010).

However, through advertising, music, books and magazines, stereotypical beliefs, and urban myths (such as boys are better at math), we've been conditioned to believe that we are vastly different—even from different planets—and that our differences are rooted in biology (APA 2005). Women are more likely to attribute gender differences to social expectations, whereas men generally believe that the differences are biological (Parker, Menasce Horowitz, and Stepler 2017). The belief in biological differences between men and women perpetuates myths about innate abilities, which justifies sexism. For instance, sexist myths influence how we treat each other: from birth, babies are labeled as either boys or girls, setting up expectations for how we should parent them, how they will dress, what sports they will and should play, and what subjects they will excel in at school. Putting people into two overly simplistic categories prevents us from seeing people as three-dimensional individuals, making it difficult to truly understand one another. Maintaining this strict binary also legitimizes inequality as natural and inevitable. Furthermore, when we categorize men and women as distinctly different, it gives us permission to forget or ignore just how much we have in common and how much our characteristics overlap (Zell, Krizan, and Teeter 2015).

Understanding the Gender Binary

Assuming that men and women are vastly and biologically different automatically places us in different camps, creating a binary system of male versus female. But consider a situation where an individual, who was raised as a female and identifies as female, finds out as an adult that she has XY chromosomes, which explains her infertility. Genetically she can be identified as male, but she looks and feels female. Is there a place for her in a binary system?

ACTIVITY: Consider Your Traits

One way to think about gender with more nuance is to consider your own traits and characteristics. Look at these traits that are commonly associated as masculine or feminine. Check off the traits that you identify with, and be sure to consider context as you do this. For example, while you might not identify yourself as generally aggressive or emotional, are there situations where you might be? Add any traits not listed that you associate with yourself.

Your	Masculine traits	Your	Feminine traits
	Independent		Dependent
	Aggressive		Passive
	Competitive		Collaborative
	Strong		Soft
	Unemotional		Emotional
	Leader		Follower
	Protector		Nurturer
	Action-oriented		Indecisive
	Logical		Verbal
	Ambitious		Caretaker

Which traits do you value more, and why?

_____

_____

_____

_____

You most likely have some traits that fall under the category of feminine and other traits that fall under the category of masculine. In fact, if you consider context, you might find that you have all of these traits! How we separate traits by gender has more to do with social expectations than how people really are.

ACTIVITY: Examining Social Expectations of Gender

Consider the social expectations that come with so-called masculine and feminine traits. Looking at the different traits listed in the previous exercise, what expectations of gender are attached to masculine and feminine traits? Write down your thoughts in the space provided.

Expectations of Feminine Traits	Expectations of Masculine Traits

Despite these social expectations, can you see from your own experience that gender doesn't neatly fit into separate categories? Instead, gender represents a spectrum of possibilities.

ACTIVITY: Seeing Gender as a Spectrum

To begin considering gender as a spectrum, take a look at the masculine and feminine traits that you identified with earlier. Where on the continuum of male and female do you feel your traits fall? Plot where you fit on the graph below.

Male ←——————————————————→ Female

To explore your experience of the fluidity of gender, choose a context (work, family, relationship, friends), write the context down below, and reflect on where your traits might fall on the continuum. Note if there is a change.

Context: _____

Male ◄───► Female

SEX VS. GENDER AND THE GENDER BINARY

Sex and gender are not the same thing. Sex refers to biological characteristics including chromosomes, sex organs, and hormones. One's sex is typically assigned at birth, based on genitalia and reproductive anatomy, which can be problematic as it reinforces the gender binary. Gender refers to how we interpret sex, meaning your self-concept and whether you identify as female, male, or somewhere on the spectrum such as nonbinary or transgender. Because our culture often confuses sex and gender, we learn and are reinforced to believe myths about both. Our beliefs about both gender and sex are socially constructed. *Socially constructed* doesn't mean that there are no actual sex and gender differences between people; it means that how we categorize people and why we do so is constructed.

The Social Construction of Gender

Our ideas and expectations about gender are influenced and shaped by race/ethnicity, culture, class, religion, the media, family, and our peers. All of these variables affect our expectations about appropriate gender role behaviors and attitudes for ourselves and for others.

For instance, one of the first things we do to identify a baby's sex is to examine the fetus's anatomy in a sonogram after about thirteen weeks in utero. The majority of soon-to-be parents wish to know the sex of their baby before birth, primarily for the purpose of planning and preparing for the baby's arrival (Chalabi 2015). Today, many expecting parents are engaging in a new trend: gender-reveal parties. Gender-reveal parties are meant to celebrate a baby's arrival and reveal the gender, which is based on an ultrasound. Typically, the ultrasound results are sealed and given to a third party; then with great fanfare, the results are opened, and the parents and guests find out about the baby's "gender," which is then celebrated. Soon after the gender- reveal party, planning and preparing for the baby's arrival include choosing names, painting a nursery, and purchasing baby clothes and toys, all of which can reinforce gender stereotypes even before the baby is born. Note that even the concept of a gender-reveal party confuses gender with sex. Gender-reveal parties don't actually reveal gender; what they reveal is what society thinks gender is, which is your assigned sex based on anatomy, and they also reveal how we expect the baby to be treated.

ACTIVITY: What Gifts Would You Give?

Imagine that you have just attended a gender-reveal party for twins where the gender was revealed as a boy and a girl. Keeping in mind that the parents of the twins expect some kind of traditional or typical gifts. What kind of toys might you purchase for each child? If you purchase clothes, what color? How about stuffed animals or blankets? Will one child receive a certain gift and not the other? Will the color of the item make a difference?

Write your answers down inside each box.

"Girl" baby	"Boy" baby

What did your answers reveal in terms of how we create gender expectations, based on how we treat even newborn babies? Write your thoughts down:

_____

_____

_____

_____

The Social Construction of Sex

How we define and determine sex is also socially constructed. We have determined sex based on genitals, reproductive anatomy, hormones, chromosomes, and even the brain. The characteristics that we use to determine sex keeps changing, however, because of a combination of a deeper understanding of biology and changing social beliefs about what constitutes sex. Changing definitions overtime highlights how even what constitutes "sex" is socially constructed, as the definition is influenced by what is socially acceptable. As an illustration, in the Olympics today, hormone levels play a central role in determining sex (Davis and Preves 2017), but in the 1960s, the Olympic sex verification process required naked female competitors to parade by a row of female judges as a gender verification test that was based on genitals and physical appearance (Aschwanden 2016). Such gender verification tests would never be acceptable today, so the definition of sex had to change to meet current cultural standards.

WHAT ABOUT BIOLOGY?

There are biological sex differences between men and women, including one's external genitalia. But genitalia alone don't determine sex. Biologically what identifies someone as either the male or the female sex is a range of chromosome and hormonal expressions and observable traits (World Health Organization 2019), but even so, we can't clearly define a person's sex on these characteristics, because what constitutes sex is more diverse than what we can adequately explain based on the science we have (Davis and Preves 2017). We also can't rely on science alone to determine sex, without considering someone's lived experience. Consider the lived experience of the people in the following cases (APA Task Force on Gender Identity, Gender Variance and Intersex Conditions 2006):

- James was born biologically male but without a penis.

- Sara identifies as female but discovered as an adult that she has undescended testes.

- Lisa was born with Turner syndrome, which means that she has only one X chromosome instead of two.

- Mark was born with male chromosomes but has androgen insensitivity, causing his body to not respond to androgen, which results in genitals that appear female.

ACTIVITY: What If Maria Is Really Mark?

What if Mark (born with male chromosomes but with androgen insensitivity) were one of the twins in the previous exercise, where you had to choose a gift for a pair of twins. Based on the sonogram, Mark was assigned at birth as a female and was originally named Maria. But Mark never felt like a Maria. Although his genitalia appeared female, he always felt male, and even as young as four and five, he would identify himself as a boy. Mark struggled emotionally, not understanding why he didn't feel like a girl, despite everyone around him assuming he was and treating him like a girl. Mark eventually had his hormone levels checked when he was a teenager and was diagnosed with androgen insensitivity syndrome.

How do you imagine that our culture's belief in a gender/sex binary affected Mark?

_____

_____

_____

_____

If you or a family member of yours were Mark, what would you want to change about our culture to make his experience better for him?

_____

_____

_____

_____

How common are conditions such as Mark's? In approximately one out of every fifteen hundred births, children are born with a mix of female and male genitalia, or ambiguous genitalia, or internal or external genitalia that don't fit neatly into any category. Sometimes intersex anatomy doesn't show up until puberty or even adulthood, perhaps when someone is tested for infertility. In fact, some people might not ever know they fall under the category of intersex, so we can't really determine how many people are intersex. However, even the term *intersex* is a social construction—a term we've come up with to describe the normal variation that occurs in nature (Intersex Society of North America 2008). The normal variation of nature also shows up in the animal kingdom, as there are several animal species that have been identified as intersex (Mascarelli 2015).

Just like gender, a sex binary doesn't represent biology accurately. Let's consider chromosomes and hormones. In terms of chromosomes, most females have XX chromosomes, and most men have XY. But some people who are labeled as women have a Y chromosome, and some men can have two or three X chromosomes.

Putting it together: although we have been conditioned to believe that masculine or feminine and male or female are two distinctly different categories, neither sex nor gender are that simple. There's no scientific basis to support a gender binary. The general idea that our culture has debates and discussions about what gender and sex are supports the theory that both concepts are socially constructed. Although we like to label and categorize people—and even ourselves—variability and diversity are a part of nature, and both are necessary for the adaption of a species, even humans.

Sexual Orientation, Gender Identity, and Heteronormativity

Sexual orientation is different from gender and sex. Sexual orientation refers to whom you are attracted to. The term *heteronormativity* describes a presumption that being heterosexual is the norm and the most acceptable form of sexual attraction. Heteronormativity helps to promote the belief in a gender binary. Within the gender binary system, there are two genders that privilege masculinity, and this system relies on heterosexual relationships to maintain the gender hierarchy. Anyone who identifies as anything other than a straight cis-gendered female or male isn't considered normal or natural.

The term *gender identity* refers to your internal experience of gender. A cis-gender person is someone whose gender is consistent with their sex. For example, someone identified as biologically female at birth and who also experiences her gender as female is a cis-gender female.

However, a cis-gender female or male is not the default gender identity. Gender, sex, sexual orientation, and gender identity all represent a spectrum of possibilities. A transgender person is identified at birth as one sex, but their gender identity is inconsistent with their identified sex. Also, some people don't identify as either male or female, and they might refer to themselves as nonbinary, gender queer, queer, or gender nonconforming. Additionally, sexual orientation is separate from gender identity. For example, a transgender woman could be straight, bisexual, or a lesbian.

Sexual orientation, gender identity, and biological sex are all different, and they all represent a spectrum of possibilities.

ACTIVITY: Exploring a Spectrum of Possibilities

Take a look at the possibilities below, and identify where you see yourself on each continuum.

Sexual orientation:

← ── →

Attracted to feminine   Attracted to both   Attracted to masculine

Gender identity:

← ── →

Female   Nonbinary   Male

UNDERSTANDING HOW WE PERFORM GENDER ROLES

Gender is something that we do in everyday life, primarily in our interactions with others, as we perform behaviors that act out the roles our culture tells us are appropriate for our gender. Many perform gender automatically. Often, when we are doing gender, we are continuing to perform traditional roles, despite evidence that society has outgrown those roles.

Doing Child Care and Housework

Women continue to do more around the house and do more child care than their male partners, even when women have full-time jobs, because society expects them to do the bulk of child care and housework.

Veronica and Steve have been married for eleven years, and they have two boys, ages eight and ten. Both Veronica and Steve work full-time, in professional jobs. Their professional jobs enable them to pay for a babysitter after school. When they both get home after work, around six-thirty, Steve usually spends some time on social media decompressing from his commute. In the meantime, Veronica gets dinner ready and makes sure that the boys get their homework done. After dinner, Steve and the boys wash the dishes while Veronica tidies up the house, putting toys and games away. Once dinner is cleaned up, Veronica heads back into the kitchen to wipe the counters down, close the cabinet doors, and gets the coffee set up for the next morning. Next, Veronica heads upstairs to make sure the boys shower for the next day. The boys are fighting over a game, and she interferes and helps them resolve the issue. She calls down to Steve (she's not sure where he is in the house at the moment) to help read to the boys and get them ready for bed. Once the boys are in bed, Veronica takes a shower while Steve reads the newspaper. By now it's ten-thirty. and Veronica crawls into bed, exhausted. Steve hints that he'd like to fool around, but Veronica is too tired. She makes sure her alarm is set for 6:00 a.m. and goes to sleep.

As a couples therapist, I hear stories like Veronica and Steve's quite frequently. This division of labor is fairly typical for middle and upper middle-class two-parent families with both parents in professional jobs. Although family roles have changed over time, wives in middle-class families continue to do more around the house, even when they work the same hours as their husband (Bartley, Blanton, and Gilliard 2005). Steve helps out around the house and with the kids, but Veronica does more. Women typically do even more around the house after they have children than they did before, as they tend to take on the bulk of child care responsibilities, and they tend to do so without working less (Yavorsky, Dush, and Schoppe-Sullivan 2015). If you noticed, Veronica doesn't even catch a break after work, and besides managing and taking over tasks, she takes on the emotional labor of the family when the boys are having a conflict. Even if Veronica and Steve made the same amount of money, it wouldn't make much of a difference. Wives generally continue to do more around their house even when they earn as much or more than their husbands (Bertrand, Pan, and Kamenica 2013).

One effect of this unequal division of labor and child care among couples is that women feel unsatisfied in their marriage, so much so that that an unequal division of labor is a significant predictor of divorce (Frisco and Williams 2003). The unequal division of labor at home is an illustration of how myths about gender slow down progress for women. No matter how much money we make or how many college degrees we have earned, society still considers our innate talents to be parenting, cooking, and cleaning.

ACTIVITY: How You Learned Housework and Child Care Roles

Check off the tasks most likely performed by male or female family members in your home as you were growing up. You can use the space at the bottom of the chart to add other tasks that are not listed.

Tasks	Mom	Dad	Brother	Sister	Other female relative	Other male relative
General indoor cleaning (vacuuming, scrubbing bathroom, washing dishes)						
Laundry						
General child care (changing diapers, rocking to sleep, getting up at night)						
Cooking						
Fixing things around the house						
Primary breadwinner						
Coached children's sports teams						
Handling the emotional labor in the home (checking in on relationships, providing conflict resolution)						
Helping with homework						
Outdoor tasks (mowing the lawn, taking out trash, washing the car)						

Based on who did what around the house as you were growing up, what messages about gender roles did you internalize as a child? How are you enacting those roles today? Are you doing something differently from what you learned as a child? Why?

Write your thoughts down: _____

_____

_____

_____

_____

Class, Internalized Gender Roles, and Structural Oppression

Although housework is a serious point of conflict in many families, middle- and upper middle-class women can often hire domestic help to alleviate the strain of housework and child care conflicts in their marriage. Middle- and upper middle-class families have more access to quality child care options, and these women tend to have more control over their work schedules than working-class mothers do. Working-class families face additional struggles. While middle- and upper middle-class culture tends to condone women leaving work to care for their children—seeing this as a selfless act—working-class mothers are stigmatized and face harsh consequences for stepping out of traditional gender roles and are judged for being working mothers. For instance, when working-class single mothers leave work to care for their children, they are treated as irresponsible (Hennessy 2015). This may result in loss of employment and other stressors. Consider Carla's story.

Carla is a thirty-five-year-old mixed-race woman who married her husband twelve years ago. Together they have four children, all between three and ten years old. Both Carla and her husband are high school graduates. Carla has worked a multitude of part-time jobs over the years to help support her husband's income. She hasn't been able to keep a job for very long, as predictably, one or more of her children get sick and she needs to stay home and care for them. Without benefits such as personal or vacation time, Carla is inevitably let go from her jobs for her frequent absences caring for her children. Carla's bosses seem to be sympathetic in the beginning, but inevitably, they become frustrated with Carla. To avoid being fired, Carla and her husband try to take jobs with different shifts so that one of them can always be at home with the children. This also means that they both are contributing to housework and child care, but this causes Carla more distress because she believes that it is primarily her job to take care for the children, and when she can't, she feels upset. Carla is in a lose-lose situation: she feels guilty for working and guilty when she misses work because she's at home with her children who are sick.

A Different Model for Housework

Balancing work and child care among dual-career couples is challenging for everyone. However, same-sex couples, who are not bound by the same gender role rules as heterosexual couples, tend to have more communication about who will do what around the house, include more flexibility, and are more satisfied than straight couples by their arrangements (Matos 2015).

Whereas straight couples tend to take on tasks around the house that they associate with their gender (men will take out the garbage and take care of the yard, and women cook, clean, and take care of the children), same-sex couples aren't restricted to the same rigid gender roles. They are therefore in a better position to discuss and negotiate which tasks they are willing to do based on what they like to do and what they're good at.

CHOOSING TASKS BASED ON TIME AND TALENT

This chart shows how Marie and Lisa, a same-sex couple with children, divvy up tasks in their home based on time, talent, and interest rather than gender roles.

Tasks	Family Members	
	Marie	Lisa
General indoor cleaning	Vacuums and does the dishes	Cleans the bathroom, washes floors
Laundry	Does her own laundry	Does her own laundry
General child care	Bathes children Change diapers	Gets up in the middle of the night when necessary
Cooking	Cleans up after dinner	Cooks
Fixing things around the house	Helps Lisa when necessary	Does most of this task or hires out when necessary

Primary breadwinner	Both	Both
Coached children's sports teams	Coaches soccer	Takes daughter to dance
Handling the emotional labor in the home	Both	Both
Helping with homework	Helps with English homework	Helps with math homework
Outdoor tasks	Rakes and takes out the trash	Does much of the outdoor work, except raking which she hates

ACTIVITY: Changing Roles at Home

How does Marie and Lisa's division of labor compare to what you were used to as you were growing up? How does it compare to your relationship now (this can include living with roommates)? Or if you're not in a relationship, how does it compare with your expectations of who does what around the house?

_____

_____

_____

What barriers might prevent you from reorganizing the division of labor in your home? For instance, will your partner be supportive of making changes? Would you be comfortable requesting those changes?

_____

_____

_____

You can use Marie and Lisa's chart as a template to create a system of your own for divvying up tasks around the house. You can either reimagine how you would divvy up tasks in your home right now or imagine how you would like your ideal family to divide up tasks.

GENDER ROLES AS A TOOL OF THE PATRIARCHY

A patriarchal culture relies on a gender binary to create divisions between men and women, and to provide justification for a male-dominated society. Gender roles can be used to reinforce and justify systemic oppression. One example is legislation that focuses on gender and the use of public restrooms. Another example is the gender wage gap.

Bathroom Bills

Bathroom bills are legislative proposals that access to public restrooms should be based on assigned sex at birth rather than gender identity. Proponents of bathroom bills intend to prevent transgender people from using the bathroom that is consistent with their gender identity, the justification being to protect women and girls in public restrooms from sexual harassment, sexual assault, and voyeurism.

The fear is that cis-gender men might dress up as women to enter a women's room, just to harass and assault vulnerable girls and women. However, there isn't any evidence that women and girls are at risk. The evidence does support that legislation like this fuels transphobia and that, in reality, transgender individuals are more at risk of being discriminated against, harassed, and abused. Anti-transgender bathroom bills contribute to the marginalization of an oppressed group by significantly impacting a transgender individual's participation and safety in life (Wang et al. 2016).

The Gender Wage Gap

Another example of how gender roles are used by the patriarchal system to justify inequality is the existence of the gender wage gap. The wage gap refers to the typical difference in earnings between men and women in the same jobs. Patriarchal explanations for the gender wage gap can be infuriating, because women are fighting for equality in a system that is working against them. Typically, explanations of the wage gap are myths that rely on gender roles to substantiate them. These myths range from blaming women (for not being assertive or confident enough to ask for raises) to accusing women of not working as hard or not being as educated as men are to assuming women will leave their jobs to have children. None of these myths are true (McCaig 2018).

The wage gap exists because women's work is devalued, and devaluing women's work is both a cause and an effect of inequality.

There are many factors that affect the disparity of earnings between men and women, but economists estimate that 40 percent of the wage gap is due to discrimination (Joint Economic Committee 2016). For instance, progress for women at work is stalled, because despite earning more college degrees than men, women in general, and more significantly women of color, are not being hired for entry-level positions at the same rate as men. Women are also not being promoted, resulting in men holding the majority of the manager positions. Additionally, women overall have less support and access to senior leaders and managers than their male colleagues and have to deal with harassment and discrimination. Lastly, lesbians and women of color are more significantly impacted by biases (McKinsey and Company 2018).

ACTIVITY: Your Experience at Work

Use the questions below to reflect on your work experience and how the wage gap impacts you:

1. Do you make the same amount of money that your colleagues with similar work and experience and educational background make? If you are not sure, is this something you can or would be willing to research?

   _____

2. How would you feel if you made—or do you feel if you make—less than a colleague with similar experience and educational background?

   _____

   _____

3. If you do make less than your colleagues, what factors play a role?

   _____

   _____

   _____

The wage gap has a broad impact. Below are some of the causes and effects that the wage gap has on women, the economy, and society (Joint Economic Committee 2016):

- Women with an education are outearned by men with less education.

- Women of color make substantially less than white men and even white women.

- Disabled women earn substantially less than nondisabled women in the same jobs, and substantially less than disabled men.

- A lack of family-friendly policies (flexible work schedules, paid leave) prevent working mothers from having access to full-time jobs.

- Working mothers who have access to full-time work lowers reliance on government programs like Medicaid and Snap.

- The United States is the only developed country without guaranteed paid maternity leave.

- Women who are part-time workers earn less per hour than full-time workers doing similar work and typically do not receive benefits such as retirement and paid leave.

- The wage gap affects the amount of Social Security that women receive.

- Caregiving (for children, family members, and as an occupation) is undervalued in the United States.

- Leaving the workforce to raise children results in significantly lowered wages when returning, which affects a woman's lifetime earnings.

- If women made more money throughout their lives, they would spend more, which would lead to more economic growth.

- Very few women, especially women of color, hold executive positions in private companies.

- Working mothers take on more unpaid tasks at home and more parental leave from work than working fathers.

- When women enter a field that has been dominated by men, pay in that industry drops.

- Working fathers are not supported to take paternity leave.

ACTIVITY: Effects of the Gender Wage Gap on You

Write down any societal effects of the gender wage gap that you have experienced or that have affected you and your family. You can draw from the preceding list of causes and effects and also write down other impacts that were not on the list.

_____

_____

_____

_____

_____

Throughout this chapter, you learned to identify the different ways that a patriarchal system attempts to restrict your choices to express yourself and limit what you can do and how much money you can make because of your gender.

ACTIVITY: Be Yourself

Reflect on the following question and write your thoughts in the space provided.

If you could express yourself in any way you wanted without restriction, what would that look like?

_____

_____

_____

_____

_____

FEMINIST REFLECTION

In this chapter, you explored how treating gender, sex, gender identity, and sexual orientation as binary systems strengthens the patriarchal narrative that a male-dominated society is natural and just. Instead, you learned that gender and sex represent a spectrum of possibilities and that our job as feminists is to help remove barriers to equality for ourselves and others. Chapter 6 will explore how and why certain bodies in our culture are marginalized and how this oppression supports a patriarchal system.

CHAPTER SIX

The Politics of Body Oppression

"I'm not trapped by my body. I'm trapped by your beliefs."

—Janet Mock

The term *embodiment* refers to the physical representation of something. Your body is affected by your race, class, gender, sexual orientation, and ability status (Caldwell and Leighton 2018), and *embodied oppression* considers how oppression is felt and represented in your body. Embodiment is the opposite of tuning out: when you are embodied, you are tuned in to your sensations and feelings and how they are expressed in your body.

Developing the ability to attend to the feelings and sensations that are expressed through your body and naming them will help you develop a relationship with your body that acknowledges you, and the unique way that oppression affects you, while helping you stay present and grounded when you are experiencing difficult emotions. Body oppression makes us feel like our bodies don't matter, which is why it's essential to include the body while doing the emotional and political work of feminism, to reclaim your body on your own terms (Caldwell and Leighton 2018).

This chapter will take a look at why and how certain bodies are marginalized, how body oppression is a feminist issue, and what you can do to resist having to choose between conforming to society's expectations or hating your body.

EMBODIED MEDITATION

We'll begin with an activity designed to help you become embodied. The term *somatic* means "of the body," and this activity is a somatic meditation that will guide you to be in the moment and experience the sensations in your body. Practicing somatic meditation will help you become more resilient to body oppression, because when you pay mindful attention to your bodily sensations, you are shifting from a thinking state to a feeling state, which can help you regulate your emotions and negative thoughts (Kerr et al. 2013). Connecting with the feelings in your body will help you rely on your body as a resource for healing (Caldwell and Leighton 2018).

Meditation is simply becoming familiar with something. When I teach meditation in front of groups, I often begin by asking, "Who here meditates?" Usually only a few people raise their hand. Then I ask, "Who here ruminates about negative things, or thinks over and over about a conversation they had in the past or a worry they have the future?" Then everybody raises their hand. Instead of becoming more familiar with your worries, or pain, meditation gives you the opportunity to become familiar with your breath or the sensations in your body. While you are meditating, be sure that you remain nonjudgmentally curious about the sensations you experience in your body, and remember that every time your mind wanders (which it will!), just come back to your breath and your body.

ACTIVITY: Somatic Body Scan

Before beginning, find a spot where you can meditate without being disturbed. Tip: If you have experienced trauma, identify a neutral object in your space or, even better, a neutral part of your body, and if at any time you feel too much sensation, bring your attention to the neutral object, and breathe.

1. Begin in a comfortable position, preferably sitting down, with your back straight and supported and your feet on the floor.

2. Notice your breath. Try not to alter it in any way, but just be an observer. Notice your inhale and your exhale. Does your breath feel cool? Warm? Are you breathing fast or slow? In your belly or your chest? What else do you notice? Remember to just observe.

3. Begin to scan your body. Start with your feet and notice how your feet feel on the floor. If you're wearing shoes, notice how the shoe feels on each foot. Move your ankles around. Feel the ground under your feet again, then come back to your breath.

4. Move your attention slowly up your body, and pay careful, curious attention to where you feel sensations. As you move from your ankles to your lower legs, then your thighs, and up your body, pause in each spot. Is there any place that holds more tension than others? Is there any place in your body that feels cool or warm? Constricted? Light or heavy? If there is any place that holds more sensation than another, try staying there, and remember to notice your breath. Remember that it doesn't matter what sensations you notice, just that you notice them.

5. Keep moving your attention up your body and breathing. Every time your attention wanders, just come back to your breath. Make sure that you notice your shoulders, and as your attention moves, up, your jaw.

6. End with noticing your breath for a few rounds of breathing in and out.

Once you get used to doing it, this somatic body scan can be practiced anywhere. When you have the time, use it to luxuriate in your sensations. When you are short on time, just do a quick check-in. Or you can focus on where you feel tension in your body and just observe the sensations there. The more you practice, the better you will get at noticing the feelings and sensations in your body, and simply observing them, instead of reacting to them.

THE MARGINALIZATION OF BODIES

When you walk into a fitness center, health club, or yoga class, how do you feel about your body? How do you feel about yourself?

Rosie is a cis-gender queer Latina with a larger body. She'd like to join a gym but doesn't feel like she's in shape enough to even walk in the door. The other women wear cute outfits, but Rosie thinks she'll look ridiculous in yoga pants that are clearly made for skinny bodies. She's also not sure how to use the equipment and is too embarrassed to ask for help. Several years ago, Rosie attempted a yoga class, and squeezed herself into leggings and a bra top, and felt physically uncomfortable from the way the clothes felt throughout the class. She was the only fat, queer Latina in a room full of thin, fit women who were mostly white, and most likely straight as they were chatting about their husbands before class started. During the class, Rosie was out of breath several times and rested in child's pose when she felt she needed a break. At the end of class, the thin, extremely flexible, white cis-gender yoga teacher approached her and said, "I'm so proud of you for coming to class and staying to the end. I fully support you taking care of yourself by resting in child's pose when you need to. It might also be a good idea to check with your doctor before you come to the next class." Rosie felt humiliated and ashamed and swore off yoga forever. Her experience in a yoga class made her feel extra cautious about going to a gym, and how she might feel if faced with a similar, body-shaming experience.

Feeling like you don't fit in or measure up to cultural standards of size and appearance can be a shaming experience for many people (Webb, Fiery, and Jafari 2015) and for women especially (Brown 2006). Shame doesn't just make you feel bad; shame makes you feel like you are bad, inadequate, and deeply flawed. Shame is a social norm enforcer and can contribute to oppression because we might do almost anything to avoid feeling shame, including make ourselves invisible or like Rosie, avoiding situations such as going to a gym or yoga class that have the potential to make her feel good about herself and what her body can do (Lamont 2015; Pearl et al. 2017).

You can develop a resiliency to shame by learning how to identify when you feel shame and understand that the source of shame is something outside of you, and not the flaws you've been conditioned to believe you have. Ultimately, shame resiliency will develop from an empathic understanding of yourself and connection with others (Brown 2006).

Learning Shame Resiliency

You can learn shame resiliency. I created the next exercise from Brené Brown's (2006) groundbreaking research on shame resilience theory (SRT).

ACKNOWLEDGE YOUR VULNERABILITIES AROUND BODY SHAME

Learning to acknowledge and understand your triggers will help to reduce the risk that you will be taken off guard when you are triggered. You can trust your body to inform you when you are being shamed, if you pay attention to the physical sensations that arise.

ACTIVITY: Identify Your Shame Triggers

Reflect on a time that you felt shame. What was the first physical sensation you noticed? How did the experience of shame feel in your body?

_____

_____

Where are you vulnerable when it comes to your body? For example, it might be the size or shape of your body, or it might be that your body doesn't meet society's expectations for gender, or it might be the complexion and color of your skin or the texture of your hair.

_____

_____

What events, experiences, feelings, or people trigger your body shame?

_____

_____

DECONSTRUCTING SHAME

In this step, you connect how cultural expectations shape your experience of your body and your vulnerabilities about your body. Making these connections will help you to stop internalizing society's messages that can lead to your feeling like there is something inherently wrong with you.

ACTIVITY: Identify Your Shame Story

What is the earliest memory you can recall when you felt shame about your body and developed the vulnerabilities you listed above? Write it down, as if you are telling a story. You've been telling yourself this story for a long time unconsciously. Let's move it into your awareness so that you can pull it apart and put it back together with critical awareness.

_____

_____

_____

_____

_____

_____

Who in this story was an accessory to your shame? For example, was your mother always dieting, or did someone tell you to dress differently, to meet social expectations around gender expression? How did these people in your story contribute to your shame?

_____

_____

_____

_____

_____

How did they benefit from your shame?

_____

_____

What experiences have you had in the larger society that contribute to your shame story?

_____

_____

_____

What message about your body did you internalize?

_____

_____

REACHING OUT WITH EMPATHY

Shame thrives in secrecy and isolation. You can help break the cycle of shame by reaching out and connecting to others to offer and receive empathy. Empathy means that we feel what someone else is feeling from their perspective, and it is an important component to developing resiliency to shame.

ACTIVITY: Rewrite Your Shame Story

Now that you have identified your shame story—and the people and systems that helped to create and reinforce the shame you feel about your body—incorporate all of these pieces in your new story. The goal is for you to reconstruct your story to include *context*, the social and cultural forces that shaped and reinforced your feeling of shame about your body, as a reminder that you are not alone in your experience. For instance, if you experienced pressure to look a certain way, make sure that you include in your story the cultural and social expectations that contribute to your shame. Write your new story here.

_____

_____

_____

_____

_____

Share your story with someone you trust, who will support and empathize with you. If you're having trouble finding someone you would be willing to share your story with, consider finding a therapist to talk to. Write down below who that might be. Ideally, this would be someone who has similar struggles as you. After you share your story, write down how you feel.

_____

If you're not quite ready to share your story, write down why that is and what you will need to be able tell your story to someone else.

_____

_____

_____

You can also express your empathy for others by reaching out to someone you know who is struggling with their body. Make conscious efforts to be kind and supportive to others with body struggles. Imagine what it must be like for them to live in the world with their particular vulnerabilities.

When in doubt, validate. Sometimes we don't know what to say when someone makes a body-shaming statement about themselves. A powerful way to support someone and express empathy, without unintentionally triggering or reinforcing body shame, is to validate feelings. Validation doesn't require that you agree with what someone said. It means that you heard them and understand their experience and feelings.

Below are examples of statements that express body shame, with corresponding examples of validation:

Statement expressing body shame	Sample validations
"My mother/partner/friend told me I'm too fat to wear this outfit. What do you think?"	"Ouch, that sounds hurtful. I can understand why you're upset. I think what's more important is how you feel about what you're wearing. Also, there's no size limit on wearing certain clothing."
"I hate my [part of body] because…"	"I understand why you would feel that way because or we are under so much pressure to look a certain way."
"Today a sales clerk referred to me with male pronouns, and when I corrected him, he laughed."	"That's terrible. I think it was brave of you to correct him for misgendering you. I'm glad you told me, and I'm here for you if you need support."

Bodies and Cultural Assimilation

Cultural assimilation is a process of adapting to or becoming absorbed into the dominant group's culture. Marginalized people face pressure to adapt their bodies (or try to adapt) either to reduce stigma or to live up to cultural norms and the dominant group's set of expectations. For instance, you may find that sometimes you alter your body language, movement, or speech when you interact with someone with more privilege than you (Leighton 2018). Or you may alter your body to assimilate into the dominant culture, through the use of skin-lightening creams, pills, relaxers, surgery, diet, and exercise. You may do this to authentically express yourself and to assimilate at the same time; it can be a combination of things (Johnson 2018). You can use the next exercise to identify ways that you may alter or change your body to assimilate into the dominant culture.

ACTIVITY: Meeting Society's Norms

Reflect on a time when you have interacted with someone with more privilege or power than you. Did your body language, posture, or speech change in any way? Describe who that person was and how you adapted.

_____

_____

_____

_____

_____

If you have ever attempted to alter your body, was the desired change an authentic expression of yourself or an attempt to live up to a cultural norm, like conforming to a gender stereotype, or was it a combination of both?

_____

_____

_____

_____

_____

We often enact body-based norms unconsciously and automatically. To interrupt this cycle, you can choose something that you do with your body on a daily basis, such as shaving or bleaching body hair, crossing your legs, or using anti-aging creams. Notice with curiosity the sensations you experience, and be mindful of your thoughts, and emotions, as you enact the norm (Johnson 2018).

You may also discover that you hold back or restrain your body in some way to blend in with a cultural norm (Caldwell and Leighton 2018). Being more mindful of when you do this can be empowering.

BODY OPPRESSION AND VIOLENCE

Jaycee is African-American and the mother of Riley, a fifteen-year-old who came out recently as transgender. Jaycee and her husband love and support their teen but are very worried about her safety in school and other public places. She has been bullied at school for years, and recently she was threatened while on public transportation. A stranger approached Riley and told her she was a "freak" and should die and go to hell. Because Jaycee and her husband support her, and have talked to her about transphobia and discrimination, Riley was able to handle the incident without feeling traumatized by it. But Jaycee worries constantly about Riley's safety and has chronic insomnia and pain from the stress of worrying. They tried family therapy, but it was too expensive to commit to. Fortunately, Jaycee and her husband found a local chapter of PFLAG, an organization uniting families, allies, and LGBTQIA people, to attend meetings for support.

Chapter 4 explored gender-based violence in the context of relationships and sexual violence. In this section, we'll turn our awareness to the threat of violence that is based on the intersections of marginalized identities. Groups most at risk for experiencing violence are African-American, LGBTQIA, young, and poor. Marginalized groups are also burdened more heavily by violence because they have less access to resources and are often treated poorly when they do seek help (Hamby 2014).

Violence and the threat of violence maintain oppression by limiting the freedom of marginalized groups. The threat of violence means that we have to constantly monitor and be aware of our bodies to be sure that we are safe (Caldwell and Leighton 2018).

Consider these statistics:

- The FBI reports that hate crimes, against an individual's race or ethnicity, religion, and sexual orientation have risen steadily since 2015 (FBI 2018).

- Hate crimes against Jews have risen 37 percent since 2015 and account for 58 percent of religious-based hate crimes (FBI 2018).

- LGBTQIA people are the most likely targets of hate crimes (FBI 2018). Black transgender women experience the highest rates of fatal violence (Human Rights Campaign 2019).

- In 2017, 25 percent of people killed by police were black, despite African-Americans being only 13 percent of the population (Mapping Police Violence 2017).

- People with disabilities experience three times the rate of violence compared to able-bodied people (Harrell 2016).

- LGBTQIA students of color experience high rates of violence and harassment at school because of their gender expression, racial, and religious identities (Diaz and Kosciw 2009).

ACTIVITY: How Does Intersectional Violence Affect You?

Respond to the following questions by writing in the space provided.

1. How do violence and the threat of violence in your community affect you?

_____

_____

_____

2. In what ways do you alter your life to keep your body safe?

_____

_____

_____

3. How do you keep your family safe?

_____

_____

_____

4. Who benefits from your limited freedom?

_____

_____

_____

Oppression comes in many forms, including racial- and gender-based violence. Understanding how violence and the threat of violence impacts marginalized groups—and recognizing that violence is, in fact, a form of oppression—is crucial in our fight for justice and equality.

THE PERFECT BODY (ACCORDING TO THE PATRIARCHY)

The perfect body in our culture is a social construction and represents hyperideals. A "hyperideal" body is represented in our culture through media, movies, television, fashion, and even dolls "that are culturally situated as ideals" (Olds 2016).

ACTIVITY: Your Ideal Body

Consider your own ideal body type.

1. If you could have the "ideal body," what would it look like?

_____

_____

2. How did you come to believe in this ideal body?

_____

_____

3. If you strive to meet this ideal, why do you want it?

_____

_____

4. Who benefits if you try meet this ideal?

_____

_____

Few of us meet these ideal standards, but we are conditioned to believe that we must at least try. And the standards we are expected to try to live up to continuously change. In 2015, Buzzfeed released a video that demonstrated how the standard of beauty for women has changed over the last three thousand years. The next exercise uses descriptions from the Buzzfeed video of hyper-ideal body types since the 1930s, represented by models and actresses of the time.

ACTIVITY: Which Hyperideal Body Type Has Influenced You?

Check off the body types that have impacted or influenced you:

☐ 1930s–1950s: Curvy bodies with slim waists, like Marilyn Monroe.

☐ 1960s: Tall, thin, and boyish. Think Twiggy.

☐ 1980s: Tall, slim, athletic, and curvy. The supermodel era-picture Cindy Crawford embodied this look.

☐ 1990s: Thin, withdrawn and pale. Represented by Kate Moss, the look was referred to as "heroin chic."

☐ 2000s–today: "Healthy skinny," large breasts and a large butt, but flat stomach. Think Kim Kardashian. This era is also characterized by plastic surgery to achieve the "right" body.

The perfect body in our culture is typically represented by thin (yet curvy) bodies that are white and cis-gender. The bodies that are oppressed, shamed, and marginalized in our society tend to be bodies that are fat, black or brown, gender nonconforming, disabled, and old (Leighton 2018).

WEIGHT STIGMA AND THE CIVILIZED BODY

How did we begin to discriminate against certain bodies? To fully understand the roots of body shaming and oppression, and how we began to marginalize certain bodies, we have to look at history. Body shaming began when weight became a metaphor for wealth, class, and self-control in the late nineteenth century. How we think bodies should look stems from the idea that fat is a marker for inferiority and an uncivilized body. Earlier in the nineteenth century, fatness was considered a sign of wealth and prosperity, as long as an individual maintained some balance and proportion and wasn't "too fat" to appear gluttonous. People were also expected to not be "too thin," which might indicate anxiety or an impure mind. But later, urbanization and mass production of food, plus a growing middle-class economy, led to cultural changes in lifestyle as well as body size. What used to be considered an acceptable expression of wealth changed as the aristocratic class began to consider the growing middle-class bodies with disdain, because larger body sizes were no longer an entitlement of the wealthy (Farrell 2011).

The prevailing belief was that only someone who is inferior would be so out of control and irresponsible that they would allow themselves to become fat. Thinness became a marker of superior status; therefore, the wealthy, men, and white people represented a higher status. The groups of people who were most likely labeled as uncivilized because of their body type were immigrants, the poor, former slaves and anyone of African descent, Native Americans, and all women, as women were generally considered at risk to become fat at any time. Women were expected to exert enough self-control and willpower to prevent themselves from becoming fat and to maintain their attractiveness for men. Even first wave feminists tried to present thin white bodies as evidence that they were evolved enough to earn the right to vote (Farrell 2011). In the late nineteenth and twentieth centuries, the ideal body type for women was tall, slender, and voluptuous. To achieve the hyperideal beauty standard, women used corsets and hoops under skirts to create a shapely silhouette (Howard 2018). Later they used girdles to create the illusion of a small waist.

Weight stigma embodies sexism, racism, classism, heterosexism, and ableism. Since the nineteenth century, white, male, able, gender-conforming thin bodies are considered the norm, the standard to which we should all aspire. This is especially true for women, who must constantly strive to achieve or maintain thinness to live up to hyperideal beauty standards so as to prove our worthiness. Weight stigma reinforces the oppression of social groups by using bodies to create a social order (Farrell 2011). This is still apparent today in diet culture.

Diet Culture

Diets are pervasive in our culture and a popular way we try to adapt our bodies to meet cultural norms. Although men face fat-shaming too, women are primarily the targets of diet culture.

Women and girls especially tend to internalize cultural standards and, as a result, see our bodies and judge them through the eyes of the culture that is shaming us (Fredrickson and Roberts 1997).

Diet culture is a system that values thinness over health. Diet culture is covert and insidious and perpetuates the myth of the perfect civilized body as white, thin, shapely, and cis-gender. We receive messages from diet culture in magazines, television, movies, and social media, in the bodies of celebrities, at the gym, in yoga class, and through our own family and our colleagues at work. Diet culture tells us is that thin is good and fat is bad, and all we have to do to be good is to be thin. To be thin, we have to maintain the willpower to exercise regularly and restrict food. Diet culture tells us that once we're thin, we will be happy, healthy, and perfect.

There are other paradigms in which to view body size, like the health at every size model (HAES), which considers body size as another aspect of human diversity, like sex, gender, sexual orientation, and race, and emphasizes intuitive eating. But the prevailing theory about weight in our culture is that fat is a disease, caused primarily by a lack of will power, which supports weight stigmatization (Paradis, Kuper and Reznick 2013). This is the model that diet culture promotes.

ACTIVITY: Diet Culture Messages

Below are some diet culture messages. Check off the messages that are familiar to you:

- ☐ It's better to be thin, no matter what.

- ☐ Thin means you're healthy.

- ☐ There are good foods and bad foods.

- ☐ There is a perfect body type: thin and toned.

- ☐ Losing weight will make you happy.

- ☐ Losing weight automatically improves your health.

- ☐ You should not trust your body.

- ☐ Your real life will begin when you lose weight.

Diet culture is ingrained in our society through advertising, social media, and our culture's obsession with thinness. Sometimes diet culture language and messages sneak up on us, along with the sexist, classist, and racist messaging that are rooted in nineteenth and twentieth century body ideals.

ACTIVITY: Recognizing Diet Culture

Below is a list of red flags that you may be exposed to or participating in diet culture. Check off any that are familiar to you.

☐ Relying on before-and-after pictures as indicators of health

☐ Referring to yourself as "being good" when restricting food and "bad" when eating certain foods

☐ Feeing anxious about food and eating

☐ Following diets with strict rules about food and eating

☐ Feeling guilty about cheating on your diet

☐ Congratulating someone when they lose weight

☐ Spending large amounts of time tracking your calories, macros, and so on

☐ Following diets or food gurus who deem ethnic food bad or unhealthy in favor of foods or diets more likely associated with white culture or privileged groups

☐ Exercising so you can eat

☐ Lack of diversity in body shape, size, race, gender expression, and sexual orientation in the marketing of your diet or fitness program

☐ Eating "clean"

☐ Detoxing to "jump start health"

☐ Avoiding exercise because it might make your muscles bigger

☐ Paying attention to marketing that suggests a specific diet is a lifestyle

For most people, a successful diet is one in which they lose weight but don't gain it back (Mann 2015). Has this been the outcome for you when you have dieted in the past?

ACTIVITY: How Many Diets Have You Tried?

To get a sense of how prevalent dieting is in our culture, and how it has affected you, take a look at this list of popular diets from the last thirty years. Check off the ones that you've tried. What was your experience? Write about your experience in the space to the right of any diet you have tried. Also name any other diets that you've tried and what your experience was.

Popular Diet	Your Experience
☐ Weight Watchers	
☐ Low carb/Atkins diet	
☐ Zone diet	
☐ Mediterranean diet	
☐ Whole 30	
☐ Paleo diet	
☐ Raw food diet	
☐ South Beach diet	
☐ Macrobiotic	

Popular Diet	Your Experience
☐ Vegan	
☐ High fiber diet	
☐ Nutrisystem	
☐ Cabbage soup diet	
☐ Grapefruit diet	
☐ Counting calories	
☐ Low-fat diet	
☐ Intermittent fasting	
☐ Ketogenic diet	
☐ Master cleanse	
☐ Other diet	

Take a look at the results from your experience of dieting. Are there any patterns? For instance, how often have you dieted? Did you lose weight? If so, how much? Did you keep the weight off or put it back on? Write what you've learned about your diet patterns.

_____

_____

_____

_____

If you are like most dieters, you've lost weight on a diet and then gained it back again within a few years. Few people lose weight from dieting and manage to keep it off. Many dieters tend to lose the same five to ten pounds multiple times. Diets are ineffective for a number of reasons, as complex psychological and biological processes ensure diets don't work. For instance, gaining weight after a diet is your body's survival response kicking in after restricting food (Mann 2015). But diet culture doesn't tell you that diets don't work; in fact, it is banking its seventy billion dollar industry on your believing that you must be thin, that diets work, and that when your diet fails, you will blame yourself, feel ashamed, and start over again. This never-ending cycle is meant to keep you in a state of shame and stress. In this state, you are unable to see that you are participating in a patriarchal system intended to maintain a social hierarchy.

Eating Disorders, Dieting, and Body Oppression

Eating disorders are complex and serious illnesses that are caused by a variety of factors that include a genetic component. Dieting and diet culture don't cause someone to develop an eating disorder, but for some people, restricting and eliminating food is a trigger that causes disordered eating patterns that can lead to an eating disorder. Disordered eating behaviors include extreme elimination diets, the use of laxatives, and overexercising to compensate for eating. Most at risk for eating disorders are teenage girls and young adult women who most likely have a genetic predisposition and biological vulnerabilities (National Task Force on the Prevention and Treatment of Obesity 2000). Other risk factors can include a history of trauma, body image dissatisfaction, and media usage (Haines and Neumark-Sztainer 2006). Social media and magazines have been found to lead to self-objectification and comparison of your appearance to others, which leads to body image concerns and feeling negative about your body (Fardouly et al. 2015).

DIVERSIFY YOUR SOCIAL MEDIA

We may not be able to control all the media images we are exposed to, but we can choose who to follow on social media. A simple yet effective way to make sure that the images you see on social media don't contribute to negative body image or social comparison is to make sure that you follow accounts that reflect diversity. Start deleting or unfollowing accounts that contribute to unrealistic beauty or body standards. Choose instead to follow accounts that present a wide range of body shapes, sizes, races, ages, gender expressions, and sexual orientations.

FEMINIST REFLECTION

In this chapter, you explored how bodies are oppressed in our culture. Body shame intersects with racism, sexism, classism, homophobia, and ableism, and these groups are shamed and stigmatized for not meeting an impossible standard. Body oppression is a feminist issue because it maintains inequality among groups in our culture, arbitrarily assigning privilege and power to white, able-bodied cis-gender males. To resist body oppression, you have learned skills to stay present during difficult emotions, strengthened your shame resiliency, and learned to reach out to others with empathy and for connection.

CHAPTER SEVEN

Sexual and Reproductive Justice

"Reproductive justice is not a label—it's a mission. It describes our collective vision: a world where all people have the social, political, and economic power and resources to make healthy decisions about gender, bodies, sexuality, reproduction, and families for themselves and their communities. And it provides an inclusive, intersectional framework for bringing that dream into being."

—Jessica González-Rojas and Kierra Johnson

Typically, when thinking about reproduction, what comes to mind is biology—including conception, pregnancy, childbirth, and the prevention of diseases and disorders. When looking at reproduction from a feminist perspective, historically our focus has been primarily on abortion and our rights to access one. This chapter, however, will look at reproduction through a much broader lens. Instead of focusing primarily on the function of the reproduction system, or exclusively abortion rights, we will use a more holistic approach to look at how nonbiological issues can affect your reproductive choices, which include parenting and sexual expression (Ross and Solinger 2017). This chapter will focus on the role inequality plays, and how it affects your choices and decision making, and how public policies can limit or expand your options (Ross 2017). Sexual and reproductive justice is a feminist issue, because without the ability to control our reproduction, and express our sexuality safely and freely, we do not have equality.

How do nonbiological factors influence our choices? When we make personal decisions, to what extent does the government, society, and our community support our decisions? Below is an activity to help you apply these questions to your own life.

ACTIVITY: Build Your Family

Reflect on your identity and life experiences and consider the following questions:

Have you been able to build the family that you want, on your own terms? Note that in this case, the word "family" can mean whatever you want it to mean.

_____

_____

What support systems and resources do you have access to that will help you build the family you want? Consider your relationships, social institutions, and circumstances that will support you.

_____

_____

What obstacles might you face in building your family, on your terms?

_____

_____

REPRODUCTIVE AND SEXUAL HEALTH IS INTERSECTIONAL

Camila is a thirty-four-year-old Latina woman with three children and in the process of a divorce. Her husband was abusive and has an alcohol problem and does not work. Camila supports her children mostly on her own with a little help from her family. Camila is poor, and she and her children live in a low-income rural area within a Southern state that recently defunded women's health care. Camila has diabetes and high blood pressure and can't take the birth control pill. Like millions of Americans, Camilla uses Medicaid to cover her health care, and although her state expanded Medicaid to allow IUDs as a contraception, the hospital where she had her last child didn't offer her one. She found out she is pregnant with her fourth child; her soon to be ex-husband is the father. Camila is religious and believes that abortion is *a sin, but right now, she is having trouble feeding the children she has, and she doesn't know how she will be able to take care of another child. She considered adoption, but how would she explain giving the child away to her existing children? Plus, she has a close friend who grew up in the foster care system, and Camila knows how difficult her friend's childhood was, moving from family to family, often several times a year. Camila asks around about abortion services and finds out the clinic that was close by is now closed permanently and that the nearest provider is located two hundred miles away. She doesn't know how she will get there and back, or even pay for an abortion, since Medicaid in her state doesn't cover it. A friend recommends that she take out a payday loan, and even though they charge exorbitant interest rates, Camila tells herself she has to think practically—after all, the interest she will have to pay back will be expensive but will still be cheaper than having another child. But Camila also feels guilty about just considering an abortion and, because of her guilt, avoids going to church, even though the church has been a source of support in the past, as she and her children have been able to access the food pantry and use the church's emergency fund to help pay their rent.*

Everyone needs different resources based on their identity and life circumstances. Camila's experience demonstrates how poverty and violence against women intersect with challenges such as lack of access to women's health care and contraception, which affect her options and limit her choices. She is also experiencing a conflict in values, as she has to choose between her religion and reproductive rights. Although we typically associate reproductive choice with feminism, when considering Camila's experience, she clearly doesn't have choices. Forced to consider an abortion because she is too poor to have another child is not a choice. Additionally, if she can't have an abortion because it is not accessible to her, that too is not a choice.

This chapter will unpack some of the issues with which Camila is wrestling, but first let's move on to a related topic: how your values play in your own decision making around sexual and reproductive health. Additionally, consider that although it may seem that reproductive issues are exclusively women's issues, trans and nonbinary people can get pregnant too.

HOW YOUR VALUES IMPACT YOUR CHOICES

Values are the beliefs that you hold that influence and motivate you to act a certain way. Values give meaning to and shape your life, as you express what is important to you in the choices that you make, how you react to life situations, how you express yourself, how you create relationships, and what makes you happy. Your values can change over time too, as you grow and develop throughout your life. Your values can also be affected by context: what is important in one situation may not be as important in another. When you make choices that don't reflect your values, you can be deeply affected by shame or guilt. Sometimes your values can conflict with your family's values and societal values, too. Life experiences often challenge us as we are confronted with decisions that reveal where value conflicts lie.

Knowing what your values are and how they can change can help you make decisions and create meaning in your life. You may already be familiar with your values in terms of your career, or even relationships. But how aware are you of your values when it comes to making decisions about your reproductive health and sexual autonomy?

Here are some examples of values that could affect your decision making:

Privacy	Loyalty	Citizenship	Risk taking
Religion	Tradition	Fairness	Well-being
Flexibility	Commitment	Curiosity	Balance
Spirituality	Competence	Contribution	Peace
Equality	Competition	Boldness	Relationships
Freedom	Helpfulness	Compassion	Challenge
Achievement	Kindness	Determination	Diversity
Collaboration	Leadership	Happiness	Knowledge
Family	Obedience	Security	Leadership
Democracy	Wisdom	Adaptability	Humility
Friendship	Open-mindedness	Assertiveness	Honesty
Community	Personal development	Altruism	Simplicity
Health	Persistence	Confidence	Self-Control
Love	Purity	Decisiveness	Motivation
Integrity	Respect for others	Determined	Success
Diversity	Respect for self	Ethical	Stability
Autonomy	Wealth	Integrity	Proactivity
Dependability	Responsibility	Happiness	Expressiveness
Sensitivity	Safety	Prepared	Motivation
Civil rights	Fairness	Separation of church and state	Self-determination

ACTIVITY: Identify Your Sexual and Reproductive Values

Read the following scenarios and think about how you might feel if it were you in these situations. Then choose two or three values that would be most important to you, considering how you might respond to these situations. You can use the previous values list as a guide, but feel free to include values not listed.

Note: Some of the following scenarios might be familiar to you, while others may seem farther afield. If the latter is the case, try to imagine yourself in this situation, and use it as an opportunity to understand the complexity of reproductive and sexual health and to foster empathy for the struggles people face that might be different than yours.

1. You are going to start a new sexual relationship and would like to prevent pregnancy and sexually transmitted infections (STIs).

   Values: _____

2. You are in a sexual relationship and already have a child and would like to wait to have another.

   Values: _____

3. You are a transgender man and are able to become pregnant, but don't want to.

   Values: _____

4. You are a teenager and feel invisible because your school's sex education program does not include information relevant to you as a member of the LGBTQIA community.

   Values: _____

5. You want to have another child, but you can't afford to.

   Values: _____

6. You have children, are poor, and live in a neighborhood where there is ongoing violence.

   Values: _____

7. You are a parent living in an urban area without access to clean drinkable water.

   Values: _____

8. You are postmenopausal and would like an HIV test.

   Values: _____

9. You are disabled but still sexual. You would like information about birth control.

   Values: _____

Write down all of the values that you identified as important to you in these scenarios, and then write a number next to each one to rank these values in order of importance.

_____

_____

_____

_____

Write the first five down in the left-hand column of the table below. In the right-hand column, turn each value into an action. Follow my example below:

Top Five Values	Write your value as an action.
Example: Integrity	Live with integrity.
1.	
2.	
3.	
4.	
5.	

Your values express your deepest beliefs, and reproductive and sexual health decisions represent some of the most personal decisions you will make in your life. You should be able to make these decisions, based on your circumstances, without interference from oppressive laws and policies, and other inequalities that limit your options. Use your values to help motivate you to be invested in your reproductive and sexual health rights and the rights of people in your community and social group. Keep these values in mind as you read through the rest of this chapter.

REPRODUCTIVE AND SEXUAL OPPRESSION

Reproductive and sexual oppression refers to social, economic, and institutional strategies and policies that limit the reproductive ability and sexual autonomy of marginalized groups (ACRJ 2005). Below are some examples of historical and current policies and strategies that oppress and control marginalized women and their families

- The control of black women's fertility and separation of families during slavery (ACRJ 2005)

- Eugenics programs in the 1900s to limit and control "undesirable" populations, including Native Americans, people of color, immigrants, low income women, unmarried mothers, incarcerated, disabled, and mentally ill women. Coerced contraceptive use and sterilization still occurs today (ACRJ 2005; Ko 2016).

- Conversion therapies that attempt to change a person's sexual orientation (ACRJ 2005) Refusal by adoption agencies to allow LGBTQIA families to adopt or foster children

- Separation of migrant families seeking refuge at the border, deporting the parents, and placing the children in the US foster care system

- States that allow pharmacists to deny women contraception

- Pregnant and laboring incarcerated women kept in shackles (ACLU 2019)

- Legislation (the Hyde Amendment) that prohibits Medicaid from covering abortion services, except in cases of rape or incest. This legislation overwhelmingly affects low-income women.

Policies that contribute to reproductive and sexual oppression maintain the marginalized status of vulnerable groups. Many of these oppressive policies are dehumanizing; imagine trying to give birth to a child in jail while being shackled, followed by having your infant removed from your care before being able to hold them? Oppressive polices that separate parents from their children are human rights violations with lifelong consequences. Additionally, oppressive sexual and reproductive policies limit the agency of individuals and groups, preventing them from making important personal decisions for themselves and their families.

ADDRESSING REPRODUCTIVE AND SEXUAL OPPRESSION

Challenging reproductive oppression means making sure that everyone has access to the same resources, with the goal being that everyone has the social, political, and economic power to make healthy decisions about their gender, bodies, and sexuality (ACRJ 2005). Three feminist frameworks can be used to address reproductive and sexual oppression. An overview of these frameworks follows, and the rest of the chapter will explore your experience and understanding of each (ACRJ 2005; Ross and Solinger 2017):

Reproductive and Sexual Health Care

The reproductive and sexual health care framework is focused on ensuring woman have access to services and information. The goals within this model are to expand health care services, research, and access to services focused primarily on preventing pregnancy and STIs. You are probably most familiar with sexual and reproductive health through your experience accessing services designed to maintain your health.

ACTIVITY: What Sexual and Reproductive Services Have You Used?

Check off any reproductive health services that you use or have used:

- ☐ Contraception

- ☐ Cervical screenings

- ☐ STI screenings

- ☐ Pregnancy testing

- ☐ HIV counseling and testing

- ☐ Treatment options for menopause

☐ Breast cancer screening

☐ Abortion

☐ Counseling for pregnant teens

☐ Infertility treatment and prevention

☐ Screening for gender-based violence

☐ Sexual health information

☐ Pre- and post-natal care

☐ Human papillomavirus (HPV) vaccines

☐ Comprehensive sex education

Check off where you tend to receive direct reproductive and sexual health services.

☐ Community health centers, like Planned Parenthood

☐ Private doctor's office

☐ School-based health center or program

☐ Family-planning clinic

☐ Other _____

☐ Have not received any services

If you have not received any or most of the services above, reflect on the reasons why:

☐ You did not have health insurance.

☐ You did not have access to a reproductive health center (for example, the center was too far away, none in your area, or you are disabled).

☐ You were not referred to or offered services.

☐ You are undocumented and do not have access to health care or Medicaid.

☐ You have had your concerns about your health and/or pain dismissed so many times, you stopped seeking care.

How has your ability or inability to receive reproductive health services impacted your life?

_____

_____

_____

Sexual and Reproductive Health Rights

The sexual and reproductive health rights framework focuses on making sure that your legal rights to access reproductive and sexual health services are protected (Ross and Solinger 2017). The table in the next exercise summarizes some of the relevant laws and Supreme Court decisions that support your rights to have children or not have children and to access sexual and reproductive health services. These decisions give us the right to privacy, the freedom to make personal decisions that affect our lives, and freedom from governmental control over our decisions.

ACTIVITY: Impact of Supreme Court Decisions on You

Read about each decision, and in the third column, reflect on how it has affected your life.

Case	Summary	Impact on your life
Skinner v. Oklahoma (1942)	Prior to this case, Oklahoma law allowed sterilization of criminal offenders. _Skinner_ established the right to have children as a fundamental right, as mandatory sterilization deprives some people and not others the right to reproduce, which violates the Equal Protection Clause.	

Griswold v. Connecticut (1965)	Established the right for married couples to use contraception as a right to privacy issue	
Eisentstadt v. Baird (1972)	Established the right to use contraception for unmarried men and women, also as a privacy issue	
Roe v. Wade (1973)	Extended right to privacy to women's right to choose, with a doctor's permission, to have an abortion during the first trimester. In the second trimester, the state may regulate but not prohibit abortions, and in the third trimester, the state may regulate and prohibit abortions.	
Planned Parenthood of Southeastern Pennsylvania v. Casey (1992)	States requiring husband notification are placing an undue burden, or obstacle, in the path of a woman seeking an abortion. Minors can still be required to obtain consent.	

The sexual and reproductive health rights framework is focused primarily on ensuring that abortion remains a legal option for women in the United States. Although abortion is the most controversial reproductive right, the majority of Americans support abortion as an option in most cases (Pew Research Center 2018), and it's a common procedure, as nearly one in four women will have an abortion by the age of forty-five. Most women who have an abortion are mothers and are affiliated with a religion (Jones and Jerman 2017). Legal abortion is a medical procedure that is considered safer than childbirth (Raymond and Grimes 2012), and the majority of abortions in the United States are performed during a woman's first trimester (ACOG 2014).

The rates of abortion have declined significantly, and rates are at the lowest since *Roe v. Wade* (Jatlaoui et al. 2018). Unfortunately, abortion has become a political issue, and much of the information presented about abortion in politics is misinformation and propaganda. For instance, "partial birth abortion" and "late-term abortion" are not actual medical terms but are political language used to frame abortion in a negative light. In actuality, second and third trimester abortions are rare and performed when the life of the mother or fetus is in danger. Some women who have had abortions beyond the first semester reported barriers to receiving abortion care earlier, such as not having access to services or being unable to pay for an abortion (Guttmacher Institute 2017).

Feminists consider the right to choose an abortion essential in the path to equality because the ability to control when or whether to have children gives us control over our bodies, our future, and our destiny. But the idea of "choice" doesn't include everyone, particularly marginalized women who, because of structural oppression, have limited choices. Additionally, an exclusive focus on abortion rights neglects the history and effects of forced sterilization in many communities. These limitations are addressed in the reproductive and sexual justice framework, covered in the next section.

ACTIVITY: Speak About Your Experience

Abortion is a safe and normal medical procedure that has been stigmatized, shaming women for their personal decision and accessing medical care. If you have had an abortion, a pregnancy scare and considered abortion, or have someone close to you with these experiences, you can push back against the stigma and shame by telling your story. Even if you are not ready to share your story with another person, start by writing it down. You always have the option of sharing your story when the time is right.

_____

_____

_____

_____

_____

Reproductive and Sexual Justice

It's not enough to have access to contraception and abortion, if your choices are limited because of circumstances and limited access to resources, as Camila's story illustrated. The concept of reproductive justice was created by women of color, based on their lived experiences and their frustration with white feminist's singular focus on abortion as the primary issue in terms of reproductive rights.

Access to safe legal abortion can't be divorced from other needs, such as education, good-paying jobs, housing, and safe neighborhoods. The reproductive and sexual justice framework shifts the focus away from the concept of "choice" in reproduction, to consider context. Reproductive and sexual justice focuses on ensuring accessibility for everyone. The framework of reproductive justice is intersectional and created to make sure that the differences between social groups don't become barriers (Ross and Solinger 2017).

By addressing systemic oppression, reproductive justice goes beyond working toward accessibility. Activists in the reproductive justice movement connect your rights to access of services with a consideration of the ways that inequality may affect your access to these services (Ahmed and Gamble 2017).

REPRODUCTIVE AND SEXUAL JUSTICE VALUES

The framework of reproductive and sexual justice includes the following values (Ross and Solinger 2017):

- Your right to have children

- Your right to not have children

- Your right to parent children in safe and healthy environments

- Your right to sexual autonomy and gender freedom

As you can imagine, reproductive justice covers a wide spectrum of social and individual issues that can affect your rights. Here are some examples.

- Access to affordable housing

- Quality of schools

- The safety and condition of the neighborhood that you raise your children in

- Being able to afford to have a child, if you want one

- The ability to create relationships and or a family of your choosing

- The right to determine your birth plan, when giving birth

- The ability for you and your family to live violence-free in your home and community

- Being able to safely express your gender identity and sexual orientation

- Interrupting the cycle of mass incarceration and its impact on you, your family, and your community

- Feeling respected and taken seriously for being a sexual person

ACTIVITY: Identify Issues That Impact you

Reflect on reproductive justice and the social and individual issues that impact your life. Write down the issues that you are facing, and also reflect on what you might need from your community and society to address these issues.

_____

_____

_____

_____

_____

_____

UNDERSTANDING SEXUAL JUSTICE

Humans are sexual beings, and sexual autonomy is a human right (Berer 2004). *Sexual justice* refers to sexual autonomy as freedom from sexual violence and harassment, along with the right to sexual pleasure.

Below are your sexual justice rights, based on working definitions developed from discussions in 2002 with sexual health experts from around the world (World Health Organization 2006).

- To receive the highest attainable standard of sexual health, including access to sexual and health care services

- To seek, receive, and impart information related to sexuality

- To have access to sex education

- Respect for bodily integrity

- To choose your partner

- To decide whether to be sexually active or not

- To have consensual sexual relations

- To have consensual marriage

- To decide whether or not, and when, to have children

- To pursue a satisfying, safe, and pleasurable sexual life

These rights are understood along with the premise that the responsible exercise of human rights requires that all persons respect the rights of others.

ACTIVITY: Expressing Your Sexual Rights

Consider your experience expressing your sexuality and sexual identity. Have your sexual rights always been respected by others? How about by your family and community?

_____

_____

_____

If the answer is no to either question, reflect on what you might need from society to ensure that your sexual rights and sexual autonomy are protected.

_____

_____

_____

_____

SEX EDUCATION AND SEXUAL INJUSTICE

A practical and profound example of oppressive polices that promote inequality between groups is sex education in the United States. Sex education is a sexual justice issue because, as a result of different policies and legislation in different states, not everyone has access to the same services. Also, depending on where you received sex education (if you did), the information you received might very well have been biased. Below are brief discussions of two different types of sex education: comprehensive and abstinence-only.

Abstinence-only programs were funded by the US government to lower the once high rates of teen pregnancy. The primary methods used in abstinence-only programs are fear and shame. Teens are told that they should "just say no" and wait until marriage to have sex. They are also given false or distorted information about sex, pregnancy, reproduction, and contraception. Instead of encouraging teens to develop critical-thinking skills and an understanding of their own values, these programs deliver the message that waiting until heterosexual marriage to have sex is the standard that they are expected to live up to. Government-funded abstinence-only programs cannot even mention contraception or safe sex. Although research does not support abstinence-only programs as an effective method for reducing teen pregnancy, many states still require these programs, and most states don't include any information about HIV either (Advocates for Youth 2014; Stanger-Hall and Hall 2011). Ironically, teen pregnancy rates have dropped dramatically over the years, nationally and in every state, in large part to more information available and better access to contraception (Boonstra 2014).

Certain populations are typically excluded in abstinence-only programs:

- LGBTQIA populations (who would be mentioned only in the context of HIV/AIDS, if mentioned at all)

- Disabled populations, as this model assumes that disabled people must not be interested in procreation and that procreation is the only goal of sex

- People who are not religious

Much of the funding for abstinence-only programs has been provided to states to use in schools that are low income and have large minority populations, particularly African-American and Latino communities. Latinas have high rates of teen pregnancies, and African-Americans have high rates of teen pregnancies, STIs, and HIV. Additionally, single mothers who are African-American have been singled out, blamed, and stigmatized by society as "welfare queens." With their focus on these populations, abstinence-only programs are arguably a form of institutional racism, as they disproportionally affect communities of color and prevent them from accessing information and resources that would help them address high rates of teen pregnancies, STIs, and HIV. For communities of color, abstinence-only sex education programs maintain racial and gendered inequality (Kuehnel 2009).

On the other hand, there are effective sex education programs. *Comprehensive sex education* is age- and developmentally-appropriate sex education for children and adolescents that is evidenced-based and focuses on reproductive development, prevention of STIs, contraception and abstinence, interpersonal and communication skills, healthy sexual expression, consent, and creating healthy sexual relationships. High-quality and effective comprehensive sex education is also LGBTQIA-inclusive and encourages participants to think critically about power in their relationships (ACOG 2014). Unfortunately, only eighteen states require information about contraception in their programs (Guttmacher Institute 2017).

Sex education is the foundation for reproductive health, and most Americans want some type of comprehensive sex education for their children, or at least to cover contraception as well as abstinence. However, even if you want comprehensive sex education, the state that you live in will decide whether or not you receive it. States determine whether they will require schools to provide sex education and often what type of program they will provide. Currently, less than half of states require information about HIV (Advocates for Youth 2014). Therefore, where you live will determine whether or not your children will have access to fact-based information about sex, consent, and contraception. Women, especially young women, in the United States have relatively high rates of unplanned pregnancy and poor access to contraception, and reproductive health services can make a huge difference in their lives (Kaye et al. 2014).

ACTIVITY: Your Sex Education

Reflect on your experience learning about sex:

1. Where did you first learn about sex (your school, parents, friends, siblings, books, movies, or a combination of these):

   _____

   _____

2. If you attended a community, religious, or school-based sex education program, did you feel like your needs were addressed in the program?

   _____

   _____

3. Did you learn that pleasure is a part of sexual health? If not, why do you suppose it was excluded?

    _____

    _____

4. Did you learn that you have a right to have sex and a right to refuse sex? If not, how might learning about these rights have affected your sexual expression and autonomy?

    _____

    _____

5. If you could summarize the main message of what you learned about sex, what would it be?

    _____

    _____

6. What role does that message play in your life today?

    _____

    _____

FEMINIST REFLECTION

In this chapter, you examined your sexual and reproductive values. You also learned about how reproductive and sexual oppression prevents marginalized groups from having access to services, and how having the ability to control what does and what does not happen to your body is essential for equality. You explored frameworks designed to reduce and eliminate sexual and reproductive oppression, and why it is key to use strategies that are intersectional and grounded in human rights values. The next chapter will explore the need for collective action and how you can become an agent for social change.

CHAPTER EIGHT

The Personal Is Political

"Service is the rent we pay for the privilege of living on this Earth."

—Shirley Chisholm

The expression "The personal is political" came out of second-wave feminism as a rallying slogan that emphasized how the personal lives of women were affected by politics and gender inequality. This book has explored how a patriarchal system creates a hierarchy, and the many ways that this affects those of us toward the bottom of the hierarchy. The effects of oppression are wide-ranging. Women experience obstacles at work, and have higher rates of depression, anxiety, and PTSD from gender-based discrimination and violence. Women experience stigma and shame from not being able to live up to cultural standards of beauty and body ideals. Some women are worried about their children's lives and whether or not they can ensure their safety. The phrase "the personal is political" is a shorthand for the connection between the issues and social problems that you struggle with in your own life and the politics and social policies that contribute to that experience. So far, this book has explored individual strategies that can help you dismantle the patriarchy in your own life. This chapter will turn your attention toward finding lasting solutions to your personal struggles by challenging social and political structures through collective action, working with others to create change (Enns 2004). Feminist activism is a crucial and consistent driver of change for women's rights, and your contribution, no matter how large or small, can make an impact (Weldon and Htun 2013).

An activist is someone actively involved in a movement to create social and or political change. The feminist identity you have developed will predict how you involve yourself in feminist activism (Frederick and Stewart 2018). That involvement will be driven by a deeper understanding of the structural forces that drive inequality as well as a feeling of connection with other women whose opportunities and well-being are affected by sexism (Swank and Fahs 2017). There are many ways to become an activist, and this chapter will focus on helping you identify the issues that are most important to you, so you can get started as an activist in the feminist movement to challenge institutionalized sexism and transform society.

ACTIVISM MAKES YOU FEEL GOOD

In addition to being a driver of social change, fighting for what you believe in through activism can give meaning to your life. Working toward a higher purpose while feeling connected to others can increase your well-being and your happiness (Klar and Klasser 2009).

> *Aamirah, an Iranian-American woman, spent part of her childhood in foster care. During the time that she was in foster care, Aamirah lived with several different families, sometimes moving three or four times per year. Aamirah was adopted when she was four years old, and fortunately, her adoptive parents gave her the consistent, loving home she needed to begin healing from her early-life trauma.*
>
> *When Aamirah was in college, she learned about reproductive justice in a women's studies class. The values of reproductive justice resonated deeply with Aamirah because of her experience in foster care. When she saw on the news recently that families coming to the United States to seek refuge are being separated at the border, and that some undocumented children are being put into the American foster care system, Aamirah was outraged. She put her feelings to use in several ways, by attending a local march protesting family separation, donating money to a humanitarian organization, signing up for free trainings and webinars to understand better the immigration process, calling her Members of Congress to complain about the policy, and volunteering to do legal intakes for a national immigration rights organization.*
>
> *Aamirah felt uplifted by her activism and volunteer work. She was able to integrate her painful experience in foster care with her knowledge of structural inequality and her desire to promote reproductive justice, to help others. In the process, she made connections with other activists who shared her values and beliefs. Aamirah knows that she can't change her story, but she would like to change policies that can help others have a different outcome.*

Aamirah's story demonstrates how the personal is the political. And it also shows how anyone can be an activist, and we all have something to offer. The first place to start as an activist is to identify the issues that are most important to you. As you reflect on the topics that this book has covered, which issues resonate the most with you? Are there certain issues that you feel more passionate or angry about than others? For example, because of my personal and professional experiences, violence against women and reproductive justice are issues that resonate deeply with me.

Getting Started

If you're just getting started with activism, you might feel tempted to work on several issues at once. You might also feel slightly anxious or intimidated and unsure about what you can really accomplish. I recommend that you choose to work on one or two issues at a time. Start with the social issues that are the most meaningful for you.

Since you'll be spending time and resources on an issue, make sure you know what you want to achieve. Consider the social issue or problem you would like to work on. What is your goal? Make sure that your goal is achievable. For instance, ending racism is a fantastic but lofty goal for any one person to take on. However, as a reachable goal, you could work on ensuring that local schools have books and programming that are focused on diversity.

ACTIVITY: Your Inner Activist

Write down the topics or issues that resonate the most with you as you consider your inner activist. What's most important to you?

_____

_____

_____

Next, reflect on why these issues are important to you:

_____

_____

_____

_____

Write down your goals.

_____

_____

A key to your success as a feminist is identifying what you can contribute to the movement. You can identify your unique contribution by remembering your feminist superpower.

ACTIVITY: Remember Your Feminist Superpower

Recall the feminist superpower you identified in chapter 3. Write your superpower down below and keep it in mind throughout the chapter. Your superpower is the unique skill that you will bring to your activism. Write down your feminist superpower again:

_____

EVERYDAY ACTIVISM

Activism can be integrated into your everyday life by incorporating the strategies in this section into your routine.

First Educate Yourself

No matter what kind of activism you are interested in getting involved in, the way to get started is by educating yourself on the topic you're focusing on. Research the social issue by reading articles, including opinion and critical-thinking pieces, and news stories. Make sure that you read pieces that support your ideas and pieces that are critical of your ideas. You will learn much more about this social problem by learning about opposing arguments. Here are some other ways to do research:

- Watch documentaries.

- Listen to podcasts.

- Research and connect with local and national organizations that focus on this social problem. (See the resources section at the end of this book.)

- Use social media to follow organizations and people who are leaders, thinkers, and workers in the movement.

- Attend lectures and events in your community that discuss this social problem.

- Gain practical experience and knowledge by volunteering with a local agency.

Choose Your Message

Once you have conducted some research, start thinking about what message you want to spread to others to have impact. Below are some examples of messages that reflect a feminist philosophy of social change:

- *My body, my choice.*

- *Pay me what I'm worth.*

- *End sexual violence now.*

- *Trans women are women.*

Your message describes the change you want to create.

ACTIVITY: What Is Your Message?

Summarize the main message of the issue that you're working on in three to four sentences:

_____

_____

_____

_____

_____

_____

Your message will have a lot more impact if you can attach a personal story to it. For instance, the survivors of the Parkland shooting in 2018 used their experience surviving a horrific school shooting to lead the March for Our Lives demonstration in Washington, DC to advocate for gun control. The story that you use to connect with or engage others can be your own story or a story from a current event or a story from someone you know (ask permission first). What is the story you want to tell?

_____

_____

_____

_____

_____

Next, connect your main message with your personal story. Make sure that it's clear and easy to share with others.

_____

_____

_____

Next, decide on a call to action. Are you asking others to take an action, like call their senator, or do you want your audience to feel a certain way?

_____

_____

Now it's time to share what you've learned. You can share your message with your circle of friends and family, share it on social media, or build on your knowledge and create blogs, presentations, and podcasts.

EFFECTIVE GRASSROOTS ACTIVISM

Grassroots activism is a movement that relies on a group of individuals to create change. A group of passionate individuals working from the ground up is an effective way to create social change, which can begin with just one or two ordinary people getting involved in an issue. A successful grassroots effort will have a clear solution and strategy in mind. While some grassroots movements become so large that they evolve into large powerful organizations, like Greenpeace, other movements create effective change based on the work of ordinary people with a story to tell.

A great example of the power of collective action and grassroots activism is the "Rape is Rape" campaign. In 2011, feminists worked together to change an outdated definition of rape. The FBI's Uniform Crime Reports, which collects statistics on rape, used to use a narrow definition of rape that was written over eighty years ago. The outdated version of rape was "the carnal knowledge of a female forcibly and against her will" (FBI 2004, 19). This version excluded male rape victims, victims of oral or anal sexual assault, and victims who were assaulted with an object. Additionally, the term "forcibly" was often misinterpreted as meaning that the victim had to physically fight back, which often led to victim blaming. This narrow and misleading definition of rape led to undercounting statistics, which contributed to a cultural perception that rape is not a real issue in our society and therefore does not need additional resources or funding to address it. The feminist magazine Ms., along with the Feminist Majority Foundation and the Women's Law Project, created the "Rape is Rape" campaign to change the definition of rape. Thousands of feminists, many of whom were everyday people, sent over 160,000 emails to the US Department of Justice, and to Robert Mueller, then the director of the FBI, to tell their stories and demand a change to the definition of rape. In 2011, Robert Mueller approved a change in the outdated definition to the following: "Penetration, no matter how slight, of the vagina or anus with any body part or object, or oral penetration by a sex organ of another person, without the consent of the victim" (Criminal Justice Information Services 2012; Feminist Majority Foundation 2012). The success of the "Rape is Rape" campaign shows how ordinary people can effect important change through grassroots activism.

Using Social Media

You can create your own grassroots movement on social media. Social media provides a fast and easy way to spread a campaign message. You can use social media to create events, spread your message, raise funds, and connect with other activists.

ACTIVITY: How to Use Social Media

Take the following steps.

1. First decide on a goal. Would you like to create a fundraiser, spread a message, or start a movement?

    _____

2. Use the message you created in the previous exercise to jumpstart your campaign. Edit your message for different social media sites, and make sure that you include your goal. Practice by rewriting your message as if you were posting on these different sites:

    Twitter (40-character limit): _____

    _____

    Instagram (300-word limit): _____

    _____

    _____

    _____

    _____

    Facebook (try to keep your message under 40 words): _____

    _____

    _____

3. Next, create hashtags for your campaign and identify trending hashtags on your topic by searching Google and Twitter. If you join in someone else's movement, make sure that you credit them.

    _____

4. Finally, post and send!

Social Activism

You can spread your message and involve more people in your activism by talking to your family, coworkers, neighbors, and people you know in the community. Social norms change when regular people speak out about issues that are important to them to the people in their lives. Speaking out challenges others to think about issues more deeply and in different ways. You can also engage or influence your community by organizing informal events about an issue. The opportunities and ideas for getting your community involved are endless. Below are some ways to get started.

- Host a letter- or postcard-writing campaign to your local or national representatives.

- Organize a night out with friends or family and make it a social justice theme: include and disseminate information about the organization you're volunteering for.

- Host a movie night and show a documentary on an issue that you're working on.

- Organize a feminist book club and offer to lead the discussion.

You can create social change within a group by convincing only 25 percent of the group's members to flip to the majority opinion (Centola et al. 2018). Start by planning what kind of informal event you would like to organize, and the message that you would like to impart to the group. If you have ten people in attendance, in theory, you only need to convince approximately two to three people to buy in to the message you are imparting, to tip the opinion of the rest of the group. You may want to host an event and invite some attendees who are on board with your message and some who might be skeptical.

ACTIVITY: Create a Tipping Point in a Group

Choose a time and place to host an event to spread your message. Use this space to write out your plans.

_____

_____

_____

_____

_____

_____

_____

_____

Become an Ally

An ally is someone who uses their power and privilege to support and advocate for a marginalized group but doesn't identify with that group. For instance, you can be able-bodied and become a disability rights ally, white and become communities-of-color ally, or straight and become an LGBTQIA ally.

ACTIVITY: How to Become an Ally

Take the following steps to become an ally.

1. **Self-reflect:** An important step to becoming an ally is to recognize the power and privilege that you have, so that you can effectively speak up for the group you are helping, and not speak for them.

From the activities in chapter 1, you have already identified the parts of your identity that have power and privilege. Below, reflect on your privilege in relation to the marginalized group you seek to help:

_____

_____

_____

_____

_____

2. **Educate yourself.** Ensure that you understand the experience of the group you are advocating for by following them on social media, reading books and articles written by them, and listening to web seminars and podcasts produced by members of this group. Be sure to educate yourself, so you don't burden the marginalized group you're advocating for by asking them to teach you issues that you can easily look up yourself!

   Summarize what you learned from your research, based on the experience of the marginalized group.

_____

_____

_____

_____

_____

3. **Decenter yourself.** Use the self-awareness you have about your privilege to understand that as a member of a dominant group, you have more power than the marginalized group. While you are using your power and privilege to help, you also need to be sensitive to the power differential. This means centering the needs of the marginalized group ahead of yours. Decentering yourself ensures that you help but don't take over.

From your research, write down the solution to the problem that has been identified by the marginalized group. Note if their solution is different from what yours was and reflect on what you've learned.

_____

_____

_____

_____

4. **When in doubt, listen.** Being an effective ally requires humility and the ability to listen and take in another person's experience. Listening validates another person's experience and ensures that you are centering the other's experience over yours.

5. **Practice.** Begin your journey as an ally by using your voice to disrupt the cycle of oppression in your own community. For instance, if you hear a family member or colleague make a sexist/racist/homophobic comment or joke, be brave and speak up.

FEMINIST REFLECTION

In this chapter, you identified the issues that resonate deeply with you, so you can begin your work as a feminist activist. Taking on the role as an activist is an essential part of your feminist identity, because you are joining a movement to dismantle systems of oppression for everyone. This chapter gave you the tools you need to begin your journey as an activist. The next chapter, will show you how to sustain your activism.

CHAPTER NINE

Self-Care Is an Act of Resistance

"Caring for myself is not self-indulgence, it is self-preservation, and that is an act of political warfare."

—Audre Lorde

Self-care as a practice of political resistance has deep roots in the civil rights movement and the women's movement. Activists in both movements recognized that discrimination and inequality prevent marginalized groups from living healthy lives. Although political power and voting rights were important during the Jim Crow era, poor African-Americans were more focused on basic needs essential to their survival, like food and clothing. White feminists didn't face the same struggles for survival generally but recognized the effects of stereotypes and sexism in medical care. Second wave feminist women of color understood from their lived experience that race, class, and gender discrimination all deeply impacted their health and survival and advocated for the inclusion of health care in the women's movement. These activists recognized that the dismantling of social hierarchies is essential to creating an environment where everyone can have access to the resources needed to live a healthy life. Self-care as a political act began when activists, particularly activists of color, claimed the right to the care of their bodies and their health. Feminists in the 1960s and 70s addressed sexism in health care by creating their own health care movement to dismantle sexist, paternalistic values in the medical field (Nelson 2015).

The political roots of self-care became diluted with the introduction of the wellness industry in the 1980s and 90s, which moved self-care into the mainstream and marketed mostly luxury self-care products. But after the cultural trauma of September 11th, the expansion of research into understanding PTSD and the broadening of who can be diagnosed with PTSD (Healy 2011) led to a reemergence of self-care (Harris 2017). The political roots reappeared with a societal shift toward taking care of yourself that has continued to grow stronger after the 2016 election, as many activists recognize the need to manage their emotions, stress level, and avoid burnout (Harris 2017).

Today our understanding of self-care and health still tends to neglect the effects of inequality and the importance of intersectionality. For instance, not everyone has access to luxury or the privilege to go on vacation, or even to take a day off from work, and a positive attitude won't end oppression. Additionally, the contemporary self-help movement's narrative is that individual deficiencies are the roots of the problem, not systemic inequality (Petrzela and Whelan 2018). This movement proposes that most of our problems can be solved if we just love ourselves more. Knowing and loving ourselves may feel empowering, but what kind of power do we actually have when we are still entrenched in oppressive systems (Becker 2005)?

This chapter will reimagine self-care as a philosophy of centering yourself in your world of caretaking. Centering your needs is a political act, because you are claiming the right to take care of yourself. And particularly when your activism is rooted in your identity, self-care is essential for you to prevent burnout and gain long-term happiness, mental health, and sustained activism.

ACTIVISM AND BURNOUT

Burnout is an experience of chronic emotional and physical exhaustion (Chen and Gorski 2015). This experience can lead to depression, insomnia, physical manifestations of stress, difficulty concentrating, the use of negative coping skills like substance abuse (Schaufeli and Buunk 2002), and feeling hopeless (Chen and Gorski 2015). Activists are susceptible to burnout because of the immense pressure we put on ourselves to create change in the world (Pines 1994) and because our emotional investment in the work is typically influenced by our personal experiences of marginalization and trauma (Goodwin and Pfaff 2001). A significant cause of burnout among activists is the belief that if we're not working to the point of burning out, then we're not really committed to the cause.

Centering your needs for self-care in your activism is necessary for your health, and it is essential that we integrate self-care as an important aspect of activism and get rid of the idea that selflessness, or working ourselves to exhaustion, is good activism (Chen and Gorski 2015). This chapter's activities and discussion are designed to help energize you, which will minimize the risk of burnout.

ACTIVITY: Recognizing Stress

How do you know when you are stressed-out or overwhelmed?

_____

What are the first signs that you notice in your body?

_____

It's important to pay attention to these signs of burnout and to address them as soon as possible. Sometimes we are so busy taking care of others that we forget to take care of ourselves.

ACTIVITY: Identify Your Priorities

Make a list of your caretaking priorities. List all of the people that you take care of and are responsible for.

1. _____

2. _____

3. _____

4. _____

5. _____

6. _____

7. _____

Where are you in your list? Who is above you, and who is below? Reflect on where you have positioned yourself and why.

_____

_____

_____

SELF-CARE FOR FEMINISTS

Within a patriarchal system, women are considered the caregivers of the world and expected to prioritize the needs of others over themselves. Challenging the status quo by centering your needs for self-care is a simple yet profound example of challenging the patriarchal narrative of women as caregivers and nurturers of other people and communities. Centering yourself doesn't mean that you neglect or ignore the people around you. It means that you make yourself a priority.

ACTIVITY: Center Yourself

Reimagine your caretaking list by placing yourself in the center of these circles, and imagine the others whom you take care of in the circles around you. Use the circles closest to you to represent the people for whom you have a strong sense of responsibility, or who are emotionally close to you, and the circles farther away to represent people for whom you feel less responsible or for work that has a lower priority.

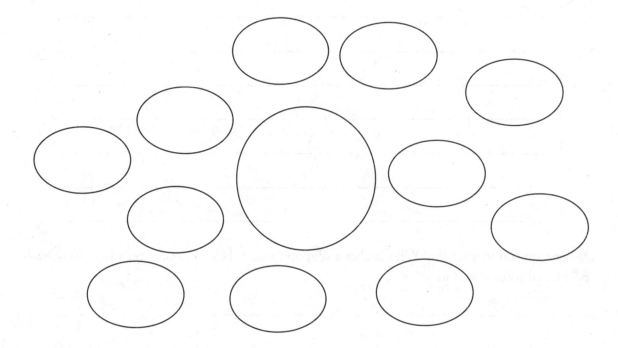

Now respond to the following questions in the space provided.

How does it feel to center yourself in your caretaking?

What might you need to change in your life to place yourself in the center of it?

What gets in the way of centering yourself?

What kind of support do you need to organize your life in this way, and from whom do you need it?

_____

_____

_____

_____

_____

_____

_____

_____

_____

What Is Self-Care?

Self-care allows you to replenish your energy, so you can continue to fight against oppression. But how do you go about figuring out what you need in terms of self-care? What does self-care mean to you?

Each of us has different needs based on our identity and responsibilities. To address self-care with nuance and an understanding of intersectionality, we can't all rely on the same definition of self-care. Instead, you need to define how self-care applies to you in your life.

ACTIVITY: What Is Self-Care to You?

In the space below, create a definition of self-care, as it applies to you, by answering the question *What do I need to take care of myself?*

_____

_____

_____

_____

_____

Now that you have identified what self-care means to you and have an understanding of what it means to center yourself, and your needs, let's look at how to do this, or how to set boundaries.

BOUNDARIES AND SELF-CARE

Boundaries are limits that separate your needs and responsibilities from others. Knowing your boundaries means learning when to say no, so that you have the energy to say yes when you want to. Setting boundaries helps you place limits on your time, personal space, and emotional energy.

Setting boundaries can help you

- Communicate your needs to others

- Avoid becoming overwhelmed

- Have more time to do the things you love (like activism!)

- Have more control over your life

- Understand that other people are not more important than you

- Feel less anger and resentment

- Create and shape the environment you live in, including your relationships

- Preserve your emotional and physical energy

Boundary setting can range from not responding to every work email to not engaging on social media with antagonistic, provocative people to determining how much of your time you will give to a cause you're working on to setting limits on your personal space, meaning, who can touch you and where. But setting boundaries isn't easy for many of us, because we have been conditioned to believe that if we don't put others first, then we are being selfish. Fortunately, it is a skill that you can develop with practice. To begin, it's important to understand that we all have the right to set boundaries and that it's up to us to communicate our limits.

The next exercise will help you begin to identify the places in your life where you would benefit from setting boundaries.

Internalize Your Limits

Review the earlier exercise in which you centered yourself. Look at your responses to the questions "What might you need to change in your life to place yourself in the center of it?" and "What gets in the way of centering yourself?" As you do, keep boundary setting in mind. Identify and write down the situations and people in your life that you need to set boundaries with so that you can prioritize yourself.

_____

_____

_____

_____

_____

_____

Knowing when and how to set boundaries is a process of identifying a problem (what you need to change), finding a solution (how to change it), and taking action. The next exercise will give you some practice.

ACTIVITY: Setting Boundaries

Use the chart to list some problems that you could solve by setting limits. Then identify the limits that you need to set and the actions you will take. As an example, I've given a common energy-draining situation for activists.

Problem	Limit You Need to Set	Action
Example: In my efforts to educate others, I spend too much time arguing and debating on social media. Although I have reached some people, it's taking too much of my time and energy.	I won't engage with commenters whom I don't know or who are needlessly provocative or are racist, sexist, etc.	I will block or unfriend people who are taxing my energy, and I won't respond to direct messages from people that I don't know personally.

Setting Boundaries in the Moment

Sometimes setting boundaries in the moment can seem challenging because we don't know what to say or how to say it. It's helpful to plan ahead, so when you need to set a boundary on the spot, you know how to do it.

Here are some basic steps. First, pause, breathe, check in with yourself and notice what you're feeling. Second, depending on what you are feeling, respond appropriately. Keep it simple: "Yes," "No," or "Maybe. I have to think about it."

ACTIVITY: Practice Setting Boundaries in the Moment

Think of a situation in which you might have to set a boundary on the spot. Write the situation down below, and how you might respond to it:

_____

_____

_____

_____

_____

_____

_____

_____

COMMUNITY CARE

Finding and joining a community of people who affirm your beliefs, your identity, and share your passion for feminism and creating change is another basic tool of self-care for activists. Activism truly is a community effort, and the real-life social connections that you make are essential to your well-being.

Here are some examples of how you can incorporate community care into your self-care.

- Volunteer for an organization.

- Join a nonviolent march or protest. Marches are effective at building momentum for a cause and giving you a felt-experience of solidarity and collective power.

- Create or join dedicated spaces that represent your identity.

- Check in with your friends and other activists to see if they need support.

- Plan or join potlucks or book clubs with your activist community.

- When you need support, ask for help from your community.

Being part of a community is essential to feminist activism. But it's also essential that you find the community that is right for you. Activist spaces can sometimes be problematic.

Self-Care in Activist Spaces

Torre does antiracist work for a nonprofit organization during most of her spare time outside of her full-time job. Torre is African-American, and this work is personally meaningful for her, as she wants to create a world that is safe for her children to live in. But the organization that Torre does activism work for is structured very much like the patriarchal culture we live in. There is a clear hierarchy of management, and decisions are made top-down. The management team is resistant to new ideas and not very open to hearing critical feedback. There is a lot of infighting among the paid staff over who and what department is getting credit for accomplishments. Some of the volunteer activists have joined in on this competitive energy and try to out do each other in terms of who is most antiracist and who will put in the most hours. Torre has also witnessed and experienced racism by some of the white volunteers and staff. The environment doesn't nurture connection or relationships between anyone, and there is little joy doing work that she started doing out of a sense of meaning. Torre experiences racism every day in her daily life and is now feeling fatigued in her activism space. She's exhausted and ready to take a step back from her activism work.

Sometimes the organizations or groups we work with and in contribute to stress and burnout by promoting the idea that we should work tirelessly and selflessly "for the cause" (Chen and Gorski 2015). These environments can become so intense and competitive that some researchers have used the term *rigid radicalism* to describe the experience (Montgomery and Bergman 2017).

This is a toxic atmosphere where activists relate to each other in hypercompetitive ways, for example, questioning who's the most radical or being hypervigilant about calling out flawed behaviors. This feeling of never doing enough and seeing obligation everywhere contributes to burnout and depletion. Activists, who tend to be sensitive to injustice, want to respond to the injustice they perceive in activists' spaces, creating more urgency and exhaustion (Chen and Gorski 2015).

Does Torre's experience sound all too familiar to you? If you are already working in an organization and realize that the environment doesn't support you, you might want to consider finding a different space that does. This would be an example of centering your self-care. If you are new to activism, use these questions to help you choose an activist space that will be a healthy environment for you.

- How does your activist space illustrate intersectionality?

- Does the culture support new ideas?

- Who is in charge and why?

- Is there a system in place to question or challenge the leadership?

- How is self-care modeled?

- What is the mood like among the activists? Is there space for all kinds of feelings?

- How do people celebrate their lives outside of the activist space?

- How are conflicts resolved?

- How is connection encouraged?

- Are people allowed to make mistakes and learn from them?

- Are well-intentioned people given the space to grow and develop?

Now that you have a better understanding of how to take care of yourself as a feminist activist, it's time to develop a self-care plan.

ACTIVITY: Develop Your Self-Care Plan

Reflect on your definition of self-care, and what changes you will need to make to prioritize your needs in your life; reflect on what already works in your self-care routine. Create your own self-care plan and refer to it when you need a reminder of how to take care of yourself. I have started the plan for you, including the essentials that we all need for self-care. Add to the plan in the space provided.

1. Make sure you eat well and get enough sleep.

2. Set boundaries.

3. Create or join a community

4. _____

5. _____

6. _____

7. _____

8. _____

9. _____

10. _____

FEMINIST REFLECTION

This chapter began with looking at the political roots of self-care. It then talked about how centering on your own needs in life can be a political act and how prioritizing yourself will benefit you. Next you worked on your own definition of self-care and learned skills such as boundary setting and becoming part of a community as basic methods of self-care. Lastly, you created an action plan for self-care that you can incorporate into your life to help you become more resilient to stress and sustain your work as a feminist activist.

As this book draws to a close, you have hopefully gained a deeper understanding of how sexism impacts your life and how identifying as a feminist can help you stand up for your rights and help you change your community. You have learned some tools and techniques to increase your resiliency and support you in your journey of identifying as a feminist. The to-do list that follows will help you locate resources to support you in your activism.

Feminist To-Do List

This list of resources will help you deepen your understanding of feminism and identify organizations that you might want to become involved with or learn more from or about. The resources are organized by topics covered in this book. Keep in mind that this list of resources is by no means exhaustive but is intended to help you quickly and easily access more information to keep up the momentum you've built developing your feminist identity and engagement in activism.

ACTIVISM

Bitch Media. A feminist response to pop culture, focused on putting a balanced face on feminism in print and online media. https://www.bitchmedia.org/about-us

Equality Now. Works for legal and systemic change to address violence and discrimination against women and girls around the world. https://www.equalitynow.org/our_mission

Feminist Majority Foundation. A cutting-edge organization dedicated to women's equality, reproductive health, and nonviolence. http://feminist.org/welcome/index.html

Indivisible. A grassroots movement of over a million members who support civic education, leadership development, legislative advocacy, and tangible action in support of progressive politics. https://indivisible.org

National Organization for Women. The largest organization of feminist grassroots activists in the United States. https://now.org

VDAY. A global activist movement to end violence against women and girls. https://www.vday.org/homepage.html

White Nonsense Roundup. Created by white people, for white people, to address our inherently racist society by calling out white friends, relatives, contacts, speakers, and authors who are contributing to structural racism and harming our friends of color. https://whitenonsenseroundup.com

ANTIRACISM AND ANTIDISCRIMINATION

African-American Policy Forum (AAPF). A think tank that connects academics, activists and policy-makers to dismantle structural inequality. http://www.aapf.org/ourmission/

Anti-Defamation League (ADL). Mission is to stop the defamation of Jewish people and secure justice for all. https://www.adl.org/who-we-are/our-mission

American-Arab Anti-Discrimination Committee (ADC). A civil rights organization committed to defending the rights of people of Arab descent. http://www.adc.org/about-us/

Black Lives Matter. A chapter-based, member-led organization, whose mission is to intervene in violence inflicted on black communities by the state and vigilantes. https://blacklivesmatter.com/about/

Incite! A movement to end violence against and within communities of color. https://incite-national.org/history/

Islamic Networks Group (ING). A nonprofit organization pursuing peace and countering all forms of bigotry through education and interfaith engagement. https://ing.org/about-ing/

Me and White Supremacy Workbook. A free workbook to help you begin antiracist work, written by Layla Saad. https://www.meandwhitesupremacybook.com/book

Racial Equity Resource Guide. A comprehensive and interactive racial equity resource guide that includes practical resources, strategies, and training curricula. http://www.racialequity resourceguide.org

Southern Poverty Law Center. Monitors the activities of domestic hate groups and other extremists. https://www.splcenter.org/fighting-hate

Women Fight Anti-Semitism (WMFA). A progressive, inclusive grassroots women's rights movement and coalition that advocates against Anti-Semitism and for the ERA. https://women fightantisemitism.org

CHILD CARE ADVOCACY AND RESOURCES

Child Care Aware® of America. Advances child care, professional development for child care providers, and works with community-based agencies to help families find child care. https://usa .childcareaware.org/

DIET CULTURE AND BODY OPPRESSION

The Body Is Not an Apology. An international movement committed to cultivating global radical self-love and body empowerment. https://thebodyisnotanapology.com/about-tbinaa /history-mission-and-vision/

Decolonizing Fitness. A platform that provides affirming and affordable fitness-and-wellness services. https://decolonizingfitness.com/pages/about-ilya

Food Psych Podcast. A weekly podcast by Christy Harrison, MPH, RD, CDN, dedicated to help people make peace with food and break free from diet culture. https://christyharrison.com /foodpsych/

DISABILITY RIGHTS AND COMMUNITY

Disabled in Action. A civil rights organization fighting for equality for people with disabilities. http://www.disabledinaction.org

Ramp Your Voice! A self-advocacy and empowerment movement for people with disabilities. http://rampyourvoice.com/

Sisters of Frida. A collective of disabled women who challenge oppression and seek disabled women's liberation. http://www.sisofrida.org/about/sisters-of-frida-vision-and-values/

DOMESTIC WORKERS' RIGHTS

National Domestic Workers Alliance. A coalition working for dignity and fairness for domestic workers. https://www.domesticworkers.org/

GENDER-BASED VIOLENCE

Amara Legal Center. Provides free legal services for individuals whose rights were violated in the commercial sex and sex trade industry. https://www.amaralegal.org/mission/

Abused Deaf Women's Advocacy Services. Provides advocacy services to empower deaf and deaf-blind survivors of domestic violence and sexual assault. https://www.adwas.org

Hollaback! A movement to end street harassment. https://www.ihollaback.org/

Incite! A movement to end violence against and within communities of color. https://incite-national.org/history/

National Human Trafficking Hotline. National antitrafficking hotline and resource center. https://humantraffickinghotline.org

Survived & Punished. Coalition to decriminalize efforts to survive domestic and sexual violence. https://survivedandpunished.org

Time's Up. Advocates for and provides legal funding for safe, fair, and dignified work for all women, free from discrimination, harassment, or abuse. https://www.timesupnow.com/home#our mission-anchor

EDUCATION ABOUT FEMINISM

Everyday Feminism's School of Social Justice. Online learning for healing, justice, and liberation. https://everydayfeminism.com/school/

Ms. Magazine. In-depth investigative reporting and feminist analysis. http://www.msmagazine.com

Unpacking White Feminism. Online and in-person workshop with Rachel Cargle exploring race, white supremacy, and racism. https://www.rachelcargle.com

GUN CONTROL

Coalition to Stop Gun Violence. An umbrella group of forty-eight religious, social, and political organizations that seek to secure freedom from gun violence. https://www.csgv.org/

Community Justice Resource Coalition. A national advocacy coalition-building organization focused on ending gun violence and on criminal justice reform in communities of color.

https://communityjusticerc.org

Every Town for Gun Safety. Americans working together to end gun violence and build safer communities. https://everytown.org

March for Our Lives. Advocacy group founded Marjory Stoneman Douglas High School students after the 2018 Parkland shooting. https://marchforourlives.com

Moms Demand Action. A grassroots movement of Americans fighting for public safety measures. https://momsdemandaction.org

ENVIRONMENT AND CLIMATE CHANGE

Greenpeace. A global independent campaigning organization that uses peaceful protest and creative communication to expose global environmental problems and promote solutions. https://www.greenpeace.org/usa/about/

350. Uses grassroots organizing and mass public actions to oppose new coal, oil, and gas projects and to hold leaders accountable to science and justice. https://350.org/about/

WEDO. A global women's advocacy organization that promotes and protects human rights, gender equality, and the integrity of the environment. https://wedo.org/about-us-2/vision-mission-2/

GLOBAL WOMEN'S ISSUES

Association for Women's Rights in Development (AWID). A global feminist organization working to achieve gender justice and women's rights worldwide. https://www.awid.org/

Women for Women International. Supports the most marginalized women in countries affected by conflict and war. https://www.womenforwomen.org/

Women's International League for Peace and Freedom. Envisions a transformed world at peace, where there is racial, social, and economic justice for all people, everywhere. https://wilpfus.org

IMMIGRATION

Border Angels. A volunteer-run nonprofit organization that advocates for human rights and humane immigration reform. https://www.borderangels.org

Immigrant Legal Resource Center. A national nonprofit resource center that works to advance immigrant rights. https://www.ilrc.org/what-we-do

Immigration Justice Campaign. Fights for due process and justice for detained immigrants. https://www.immigrationjustice.us/home

RAICES. A nonprofit organization that offers free services to refugees and immigrant families. https://www.raicestexas.org/about/

INDIGENOUS GROUPS

Alaska Federation of Natives. Statewide organization focused on enhancing and promoting the cultural, economic, and political voice of the Alaskan Native community. https://www.native federation.org

Indian Law Resource Center. Provides legal assistance to combat racism and oppression and to protect indigenous peoples of the Americas' land, culture, and way of life. https://indianlaw.org /content/about-center

Native American Rights Fund. Provides legal assistance to Native American tribes, organizations, and individuals. https://www.narf.org

Women Empowering Women for Indigenous Nations (WEWIN). Founded by Indian women and dedicated to sustaining tribal cultures, history, and inherit rights of native people. http:// www.wewin04.org

LGBTQIA

GLSEN. National education organization focused on ensuring safety in and affirming K-12 schools. https://www.glsen.org/learn/about-glsen

Human Rights Campaign (HRC). The largest civil rights organization working to achieve equality for lesbian, gay, bisexual, transgender, and queer Americans. https://www.hrc.org/hrc -story/about-us

Intersex Society of North America (ISNA). Devoted to systemic change to end shame, secrecy, and unwanted genital surgeries for intersex people. http://www.isna.org

National Center for Transgender Equality. Focuses on life-saving change and advocacy for transgender people in Washington, DC. https://transequality.org/history

National LGBTQIA Task Force. Focuses on ensuring freedom, justice, and equality for LGBTQIA people. http://www.thetaskforce.org/

Transgender Law Center. Focuses on changing law, policy, and attitudes so that all people can live safely and free from discrimination regardless of gender identity or expression. https://trans genderlawcenter.org/

MASS INCARCERATION

The Sentencing Project. Works toward a fair and effective criminal justice system. https://www .sentencingproject.org

Vera Institute of Justice. Working to improve the criminal justice system by securing equal justice, ending mass incarceration, and strengthening families and communities. https://www .vera.org/about

MENTAL HEALTH RESOURCES

Anxiety and Depression Association of America (ADAA). Dedicated to the prevention and treatment of depression, anxiety, PTSD, OCD, and other co-occurring disorders. https://adaa .org/who-we-are

Crisis Text Line. Provides free support by trained volunteers for anyone in crisis, 24/7. Text HOME to 741741. https://www.crisistextline.org

National Alliance on Mental Illness. Grassroots mental health organization that offers educational programs, advocacy, and public awareness to fight stigma. https://www.nami.org

National Eating Disorder Association (NEDA). Supports individuals and families affected by eating disorders through community education, resources, and research. https://www.national eatingdisorders.org/about-us/our-work

REPRODUCTIVE HEALTH, RIGHTS, AND JUSTICE

Advocates for Youth. Sexual health advocacy for young people. https://advocatesforyouth.org /about/

Daughters of the Diaspora, Inc. Provides programs that teach self-esteem and reproductive health to young women in the African diaspora. http://www.dodiaspora.org/about-us.html

Forward Together. Rights, recognition, and resources for all families. Reproductive justice tools and resources for all families. https://forwardtogether.org/tools/

NARAL Pro-Choice America. Reproductive rights advocacy. https://www.prochoiceamerica .org

Native American Women's Health Education Resource Center. A health and human rights collective for indigenous peoples. http://www.nativeshop.org

Planned Parenthood. Reproductive health services. https://www.plannedparenthood.org

Religious Institute. A multifaith organization that advocates for sexual, gender, reproductive health, education, and justice in faith communities and society. religiousinstitute.org

Scarleteen. Inclusive, comprehensive, and supportive sexuality and relationship education for teens and emerging adults. http://www.scarleteen.com/

Sister Song. A women-of-color reproductive justice collective. https://www.sistersong.net

POLITICS AND ELECTIONS

Dare to Run. A nonpartisan organization that educates and empowers women to run for public office. https://www.daretorun.org/

League of Women Voters. A nonpartisan political organization that educates voters, fights for voting rights, and opposes gerrymandering. https://www.lwv.org

Emily's List. Focused on electing pro-choice Democratic women to office. https://www.emilyslist.org

March On. Founded by leaders of the sister marches across the country, focuses political strategies to coordinate concrete actions at federal, state, and local levels. https://www.wearemarchon.org

Acknowledgments

Writing a book seems like a solitary activity but, in reality, requires a great deal of support from others to be able to get done. Essentially, everyone close to me had to live with my writing this book while I was also teaching and seeing clients. From serving as readers to help flesh out ideas to putting up with my sometimes overwhelm and general unavailability, my family, friends, coworkers, and students have been overwhelmingly supportive, positive, and helpful.

I am grateful for my husband, Dave, who was always ready to do whatever is necessary to support me and has even managed to teach me a thing or two about feminism. Thank you to my sister-in-law, Maureen, who enthusiastically waited for each batch of chapters.

My commitment to writing a book about intersectional feminism could not be achieved without my friends, colleagues, and students who agreed to read the manuscript and provide insights from their own life experiences. Thank you to my friend and colleague Brook Bralove, former student Joy Addae, and colleagues Jennifer Rollin and Brett Pelham for your insights, wisdom, and expertise. And a thank you to my fall 2018 semester Women's Studies 101 class for your enthusiasm, support, and very generous feedback. I promised I would name you all, so here you are: Akonor Lydia Darkoa, Lydia Dagne, Andrew Paison, Orinayo Ifaturoti, Zidane Joeseph, Ellandra Hill, Sandra Ijeoma Onwuchelu, Russell Tchatchou Nya, Alexia Hernandez, Emma Shuster, Johnny Reyes, Danielle White, Grace Esbaugh, Vanessa Rovira, Mikaela Cajigal, Saideh Saidian, Heidy Rivera, Jessica Ramirez, Dakontee Roberts, Susuana Eduafo, and Joselyn Morales.

I researched and wrote some of this book while on sabbatical at Montgomery College, and I feel fortunate to have had the opportunity to have a semester to devote primarily to writing this book.

Lastly, I would not have had the opportunity to write this book if Elizabeth Hollis Hanson from New Harbinger hadn't reached out to me to query my interest in writing a book about mental health and feminism. And thank you to my editor Caleb Beckwith and copy editor Brady Kahn for helping me fine-tune my concept and writing.

References

ACLU (American Civil Liberties Union). 2019. "The Shackling of Pregnant Women and Girls in US Prisons, Jails, and Youth Detention Centers." ACLU Reproductive Freedom Project and ACLU National Prison Project briefing paper. Accessed March 31. https://www.aclu.org/sites/default/files/field_document/anti-shackling_briefing_paper_stand_alone.pdf.

ACOG (American College of Obstetricians and Gynecologists). 2014. "Increasing Access to Abortion." Committee Opinion No. 613. *Obstetrics and Gynecology* 124: 1060–65.

ACRJ (Asian Communities for Reproductive Justice). 2005. *A New Vision for Advancing Our Movement for Reproductive Health, Reproductive Rights and Reproductive Justice*. https://forwardtogether.org/wp-content/uploads/2017/12/ACRJ-A-New-Vision.pdf.

Advocates for Youth. 2014. "Sexuality Education: Building an Evidence and Rights-Based Approach to Healthy Decision-Making." Fact sheets for activists. August 4. https://advocatesforyouth.org/resources/fact-sheets/sexuality-education-2/.

Ahmed, O., and C. M. Gamble. 2017. "Reproductive Justice: What It Means and Why It Matters (Now More than Ever)." *Public Health Post*. Boston University School of Public Health. January 16. https://www.publichealthpost.org/viewpoints/reproductive-justice/.

Ali, A., P. J., Caplan, and R. Fagnant. 2010. "Gender Stereotypes in Diagnostic Criteria." In *Handbook of Gender Research in Psychology*. Vol. 2, *Gender Research in Social and Applied Psychology*, edited by J. C. Chrisler and D. R. McCreary. New York: Springer.

Alice Paul Institute. 2018. "ERA History." https://www.equalrightsamendment.org/history.

Anderson, H., and M. Daniels. 2016. "Film Dialogue: From 2,000 Screenplays, Broken Down by Gender and Age." *The Pudding*. April. https://pudding.cool/2017/03/film-dialogue/index.html.

Andrade, A. L., Jr. 2013. "Coping with Racial Microaggressions: The Moderating Effects of Coping Strategies on Microaggression Distress." PhD diss., Roosevelt University. ProQuest (UMI 3604740).

APA (American Psychological Association). 2005. "Men and Women: No Big Difference." October 20. https://www.apa.org/research/action/difference.aspx.

APA (American Psychological Association) Task Force on Gender Identity, Gender Variance and Intersex Conditions. 2006. "Answers to Your Questions About Individuals with Intersex Conditions." https://www.apa.org/topics/lgbt/intersex.pdf.

Aschwanden, C. 2016. "The Olympics Are Still Struggling to Define Gender." *FiveThirtyEight*. June 28. https://fivethirtyeight.com/features/the-olympics-are-still-struggling-to-define-gender/.

Associated Press. 1992. "Robertson Letter Attacks Feminists." *The New York Times*, August 26, A16.

Astbury, J. 2001. "Gender Disparities in Mental Health." Mental Health. Ministerial Round Tables, 54th World Health Assembly, WHO, Geneva, Switzerland. http://www.who.int/mental_health/media/en/242.pdf.

Bartley, S., P. Blanton, and J. Gilliard. 2005. "Husbands and Wives in Dual-Earner Marriages: Decision-Making, Gender Role Attitudes, Division of Household Labor, and Equity." *Marriage and Family Review* 37 (4): 69–94.

Bates, L. 2016. *Everyday Sexism: The Project That Inspired a Worldwide Movement*. New York: St. Martin's Press.

Bearman, S., N. Korobov, and A. Thorne. 2009. "The Fabric of Internalized Sexism." *Journal of Integrated Social Sciences* 1 (1): 10–47.

Becker, D. 2005. *The Myth of Empowerment: Women and the Therapeutic Culture in America*. New York: NYU Press.

Becker, J. C., and S. C. Wright. 2011. "Yet Another Dark Side of Chivalry: Benevolent Sexism Undermines and Hostile Sexism Motivates Collective Action for Social Change." *Journal of Personality and Social Psychology* 101 (1), 62–77.

Bedera, N., and K. Nordmeyer. 2015. "'Never Go Out Alone': An Analysis of College Rape Prevention Tips." *Sexuality and Culture* 19 (3): 533–42.

Berer, M. 2004. "Sexuality, Rights and Social Justice." *Reproductive Health Matters* 12 (23): 6–11.

Berg, S. H. 2006. "Everyday Sexism and Posttraumatic Stress Disorder in Women: A Correlational Study." *Violence Against Women* 12 (10): 970–88.

Bertrand, M., J. Pan, and E. Kamenica. 2013. "Gender Identity and Relative Income Within Households." NBER Working Paper 19023, National Bureau of Economic Research, Cambridge, MA. http://www.nber.org/papers/w19023.pdf.

Boonstra, H. D. 2014. "What Is Behind the Declines in Teen Pregnancy Rates?" *Guttmacher Policy Review* 17 (3). September 3. https://www.guttmacher.org/gpr/2014/09/what-behind-declines-teen-pregnancy-rates.

Breiding, M. J., J. Chen, and M. C. Black. 2014. *Intimate Partner Violence in the United States—2010*. Atlanta, GA: National Center for Injury Prevention and Control, Centers for Disease Control and Prevention.

Brown, B. 2006. "Shame Resilience Theory: A Grounded Theory Study on Women and Shame." *Families in Society* 87 (1): 43–52.

Brown, M. J. 2003. "Advocates in the Age of Jazz: Women and the Campaign for the Dyer Anti-Lynching Bill." *Peace and Change* 28 (3): 378–419.

Buchwald, E., P. Fletcher, and M. Roth, 1993. *Transforming a Rape Culture*. Minneapolis: Milkweed Editions.

Burgess, K. D. 2013. "The Effect of Hostile and Benevolent Sexism on Women's Cardiovascular Reactivity to and Recovery from a Laboratory Stressor." *Graduate Theses and Dissertations*. http://scholarcommons.usf.edu/etd/4646.

BuzzfeedVideo. 2015. *Women's Ideal Body Types Throughout History*. January 26. https://www.youtube.com/watch?v=XrpOzJZu0a4.

Caldwell, C., and L. B. Leighton. 2018. "Introduction." In *Oppression and the Body: Roots, Resistance, and Resolutions*, edited by C. Caldwell and L. B. Leighton. Berkeley, CA: North Atlantic Books.

Callaghan, W. M. 2012. "Overview of Maternal Mortality in the United States." *Seminars in Perinatology* 36 (1): 2–6.

CAWP (Center for American Women and Politics). 2018. "Women in the US Congress." Center for American Women in Politics. Rutgers University. http://www.cawp.rutgers.edu/women-us-congress-2018.

Caygle, H. 2018. "Record-Breaking Number of Women Run for Office." *Politico*. March 8. https://www.politico.com/story/2018/03/08/women-rule-midterms-443267.

Centola, D., J. Becker, D. Brackbill, and A. Baronchelli. 2018. "Experimental Evidence for Tipping Points in Social Convention." *Science* 360 (6393): 1116–19.

Chalabi, M. 2015. "How Many Parents-to-Be Want to Know the Baby's Sex?" *FiveThirtyEight*. July 22. https://fivethirtyeight.com/?s=how+many+parents+want+to+know+the+baby%27s+sex.

Chen, C. W., and P. C. Gorski. 2015. "Burnout in Social Justice and Human Rights Activists: Symptoms, Causes and Implications." *Journal of Human Rights Practice* 7 (3): 366–90.

Chenoweth, E., and J. Pressman. 2017. "This Is What We Learned by Counting the Women's Marches." *Monkey Cage* (blog), February 7. *The Washington Post*. https://www.washingtonpost.com.

Cheung, F., C. M. Ganote, and T. J. Souza. 2016. "Microaggressions and Microresistance: Supporting and Empowering Students." In *Faculty Focus Special Report: Diversity and Inclusion in the College Classroom*. Magna Publication. https://www.facultyfocus.com/free-reports/diversity-and-inclusion-in-the-college-classroom/.

Chivers-Wilson, K. A. 2006. "Sexual Assault and Posttraumatic Stress Disorder: A Review of the Biological, Psychological and Sociological Factors and Treatments." *McGill Journal of Medicine* 9 (2): 111–18.

Cobb, J. 2016. "The Matter of Black Lives." *The New Yorker*, March 14. https://www.newyorker.com/magazine/2016/03/14/where-is-black-lives-matter-headed.

Collins, P. H. 2000. *Black Feminist Thought: Knowledge, Consciousness and the Politics of Empowerment*. New York: Routledge.

Cooper, B. 2018. *Eloquent Rage: A Black Feminist Discovers Her Superpower*. New York: St. Martin's Press.

Copeland, C. 2014. *Employment-Based Retirement Plan Participation: Geographic Differences and Trends, 2013*. EBRI Issue Brief. October 27. https://www.ebri.org/content/employment-based-retirement-plan-participation-geographic-differences-and-trends-2013-5451.

Creanga, A. A., C. J. Berg, C. Syverson, K. Seed, F. C. Bruce, and W. M. Callaghan. 2015. "Pregnancy-Related Mortality in the United States, 2006–2010." *Obstetrics and Gynecology Journal* 125 (1): 5–12.

Crenshaw, K. 1989. "Demarginalizing the Intersection of Race and Sex: A Black Feminist Critique of Antidiscrimination Doctrine, Feminist Theory, and Antiracist Politics." *University of Chicago Legal Forum* 140: 139–67.

Criminal Justice Information Services. 2012. "UCR Program Changes Definition of Rape." *CJIS Link*. March 19. https://www.fbi.gov/services/cjis/cjis-link/ucr-program-changes-definition-of-rape.

David, R. J., and J. W. Collins. 1991. "Bad Outcomes in Black Babies: Race or Racism?" *Ethnicity and Disease* 1 (3): 236–44.

Davis, G., and S. Preves, 2017. "Intersex and the Social Construction of Sex." *Contexts* 16 (1): 80.

Desai, A. D., K. M. Edwards, and C. A. Gidycz. 2008. "Testing an Integrative Model of Sexual Aggression in College Men." In Sexual Violence Perpetration: Individual and Contextual Factors. Symposium conducted at the annual meeting of the Association for Behavioral and Cognitive Therapies, Orlando, FL, November.

Diaz, E. M. and J. G. Kosciw. 2009. *Shared Differences: The Experiences of Lesbian, Gay, Bisexual, and Transgender Students of Color in Our Nation's Schools*. Gay, Lesbian, and Straight Educational Network. https://www.glsen.org/sites/default/files/Shared%20Differences.pdf.

Eagly, A. H., and L. L. Carli. 2007. *Through the Labyrinth*. Cambridge, MA: Harvard Business Review Press.

Edwards, K. M., J. A., Turchik, C. M. Dardis, N. Reynolds, and C. A. Gidycz. 2011. "Rape Myths: History, Individual and Institutional-Level Presence, and Implications for Change." *Sex Roles* 65: 761–73.

Eliot, L. 2010. *Pink Brain, Blue Brain: How Small Differences Grow into Troublesome Gaps—And What We Can Do About It*. Reprint ed. New York: Mariner Books.

Enns, C. Z. 2004. *Feminist Theories and Feminist Psychotherapies: Origins, Themes, and Diversity*. 2nd ed. Binghamton, NY: The Haworth Press.

Fardouly, J., P. C. Diedrichs, L. R. Vartanian, and E. Halliwell. 2015. "The Mediating Role of Appearance Comparisons in the Relationship Between Media Usage and Self-Objectification in Young Women." *Psychology of Women Quarterly* 39 (4): 447–57.

Farrell, A. E. 2011. *Fat Shame: Stigma and the Fat Body in American Culture*. New York: NYU Press.

FBI (Federal Bureau of Investigation). 2004. *Uniform Crime Reporting Handbook*. US Department of Justice. https://ucr.fbi.gov/additional-ucr-publications/ucr_handbook.pdf.

———. 2018. *Hate Crime Statistics, 2017*. Uniform Crime Report. US Department of Justice. https://ucr.fbi.gov/hate-crime/2017/topic-pages/victims.pdf.

Feminist Majority Foundation. 2012. "Feminist Majority Foundation Celebrates FBI Approval of New Rape Definition: FBI Director's Action Follows Extensive Campaign by Women's Rights Supporters." Press release, January 6. Retrieved from http://www.feminist.org/news/pressstory.asp?id=13402.

Fisher, B. S., and J. J. Sloan. 2003. "Unraveling the Fear of Victimization Among College Women: Is the 'Shadow of Sexual Assault Hypothesis' Supported?" *Justice Quarterly* 20 (3): 633–59.

Fiske, S. T., and S. E. Taylor. 1991. *Social Cognition*. 2nd ed. New York: McGraw-Hill.

Flannery, M. E. 2014. "Report: Time to End Harmful, Exclusionary School Discipline Policies." *NEA Today*. June 3. http://neatoday.org/2014/06/03/report-time-to-end-harmful-exclusionary-school-discipline-policies/.

———. 2015. "The School-to-Prison Pipeline: Time to Shut It Down." *NEA Today*. January 5. http://neatoday.org/2015/01/05/school-prison-pipeline-time-shut/.

Foley, D. 2017. "NPS: Cleanup 'Going Well' After Inauguration, Women's March." WTOP. January 22. https://wtop.com/local/2017/01/nps-cleanup-going-well-after-inauguration-womens-march/.

Frederick, J. K., and A. J. Stewart. 2018. "'I Became a Lioness': Pathways to Feminist Identity Among Women's Movement Activists." *Psychology of Women Quarterly* 42 (3): 263–78.

Fredrickson, B. L., and T. A. Roberts. 1997. "Objectification Theory: Toward Understanding Women's Lived Experiences and Mental Health Risks." *Psychology of Women Quarterly* 21 (2): 173–206.

Frisco, M. L., and K. Williams. 2003. "Perceived Housework Equity, Marital Happiness, and Divorce in Dual-Earner Households." *Journal of Family Issues* 24 (1): 51–73.

Gillis, M. J., and A. T. Jacobs. 2016. *Introduction to Women's and Gender Studies: An Interdisciplinary Approach*. New York: Oxford University Press.

Ginzberg, L. D. 2002. "Re-viewing the First Wave." *Feminist Studies* 28 (2): 418–34.

Glick, P., and S. T. Fiske. 1996. "The Ambivalent Sexism Inventory: Differentiating Hostile and Benevolent Sexism." *Journal of Personality and Social Psychology* 70 (3): 491–512.

———. 2001. "An Ambivalent Alliance: Hostile and Benevolent Sexism As Complementary Justifications for Gender Inequality." *American Psychologist* 56 (2): 109–18.

Goodman, D. J. 2015. "Oppression and Privilege: Two Sides of the Same Coin." *Journal of Intercultural Communication* 18: 1–14.

Goodwin, J., and S. Pfaff. 2001. "Emotion Work in High-Risk Social Movements: Managing Fear in the US and East German Civil Rights Movements." In *Passionate Politics: Emotions and Social Movements*, edited by J. Goodwin, J. M. Jasper, and F. Polletta. Chicago: University of Chicago Press.

Greenberg, N., J. A. Carr, and C. H. Summers. 2002. "Causes and Consequences of Stress." *Integrative and Comparative Biology* 42 (3): 508–16.

Gruber, M. 2003. "Cognitive Dissonance Theory and Motivation for Change: A Case Study." *Gastroenterology Nursing* 26 (6): 242–45.

Guttmacher Institute. 2017. "Later Abortion." *Evidence You Can Use.* January. https://www.guttmacher.org /evidence-you-can-use/later-abortion.

Haines, J., and D. Neumark-Sztainer. 2006. "Prevention of Obesity and Eating Disorders: A Consideration of Shared Risk Factors." *Health Education Research* 21 (6): 770–82.

Hamby, S. 2014. "Violence and Diverse Forms of Oppression." *OUPblog.* November 21. https://blog.oup .com/2014/11/violence-oppression-research/.

Hanks, A., D., Solomon, and C. E Weller. 2018. "Systemic Inequality: How America's Structural Racism Helped Create the Black-White Wealth Gap." *Center for American Progress.* February 21. https://www .americanprogress.org/issues/race/reports/2018/02/21/447051/systematic-inequality/#.Wy0rAOKBiIU .email.

Harrell, E. 2016. *Crime Against Persons with Disabilities, 2009-2014-Statistical Tables.* US Department of Justice, Bureau of Justice Statistics. November. https://www.bjs.gov/content/pub/pdf/capd0914st.pdf.

Harris, A. 2017. "A History of Self-Care. From Its Radical Roots to Its Yuppie-Driven Middle Age to Its Election-Inspired Resurgence." *Slate.* April 5. http://www.slate.com/articles/arts/culturebox/2017/04/the _history_of_self_care.html.

Healy, M. 2011. "9/11 Attacks Lead to More Study of Post-Traumatic Stress Disorder." *Los Angeles Times,* September 5. https://www.latimes.com/health/la-xpm-2011-sep-05-la-he-911-ptsd-20110905-story.html.

Hegewisch, A., and E. Williams-Baron 2018. *The Gender Wage Gap by Occupation 2017 and by Race and Ethnicity.* Institute for Women's Policy Research. April 9. https://iwpr.org/publications/gender-wage-gap -occupation-2017-race-ethnicity/.

Hennessy, J. 2015. "Low-Income and Middle-Class Mothers Gendered Work and Family Schemas." *Sociology Compass.* December 2. https://doi.org/10.1111/soc4.12333.

Hill-Collins, P. 1990. *Black Feminist Thought: Knowledge, Consciousness, and the Politics of Empowerment.* Boston: Unwin Hyman.

Hoffmann, D. E., and A. J. Tarzian. 2001. "The Girl Who Cried Pain: A Bias Against Women in the Treatment of Pain." *Journal of Law, Medicine and Ethics* 29 (1): 13–27.

hooks, b. 2000. *Feminist Theory from Margin to Center.* 2nd ed. Cambridge, MA: South End Press.

———. 2014. *Feminism Is for Everybody: Passionate Politics.* 2nd ed. New York: Routledge.

Howard, J. 2018. "The History of the 'Ideal' Woman and Where That Has Left Us." *CNN Health.* March 9. https://www.cnn.com/2018/03/07/health/body-image-history-of-beauty-explainer-intl/index.html.

Human Rights Campaign. 2019. "Being African American and LGBTQIA: An Introduction." Accessed March 31. https://www.hrc.org/resources/being-african-american-LGBTQIA-an-introduction.

Intersex Society of North America. 2008. "What Is Intersex?" http://www.isna.org/faq/what_is_intersex.

Irey, S. 2013. "How Asian American Women Perceive and Move Toward Leadership Roles in Community Colleges: A Study of Insider Counter Narratives." PhD dissertation. University of Washington. https:// digital.lib.washington.edu/researchworks/bitstream/handle/1773/22898/Irey_washington_0250E_11343 .pdf?sequence=1&isAllowed=y.

Jackson, E. M. 2013. "Stress Relief: The Role of Exercise in Stress Management." *ACSM'S Health and Fitness Journal* 17 (3): 14–19.

James, S. E., J. L., Herman, S. Rankin, M. Keisling, L. Mottet, and M. Anafi. 2016. *The Report of the 2015 US Transgender Survey.* Washington, DC: National Center for Transgender Equality. https://transequality.org /sites/default/files/docs/usts/USTS-Full-Report-Dec17.pdf.

Jatlaoui, T. C., M. E. Boutot, M.G. Mandel, M. K. Whiteman, A. Ti, E. Peterson, and K. Pazol. 2018. "Abortion Surveillance–United States, 2015." *MMWR Surveillance Summaries* 67 (13): 1–45.

Johnson, A. G. 2014. *The Gender Knot: Unraveling Our Patriarchal Legacy.* 3rd ed. Philadelphia: Temple University Press.

Johnson, R. 2018. "Queering/Querying the Body: Sensation and Curiosity in Disrupting Body Norms." In *Oppression and the Body: Roots, Resistance, and Resolutions,* edited by C. Caldwell and L. B. Leighton. Berkeley, CA: North Atlantic Books.

Joint Economic Committee, United States Congress. 2016. *Gender Pay Inequality: Consequences for Women, Families, and the Economy.* A report by the Joint Economic Committee Democratic staff. April. https:// www.jec.senate.gov/public/_cache/files/0779dc2f-4a4e-4386-b847-9ae919735acc/gender-pay-inequality ----us-congress-joint-economic-committee.pdf.

Jones, R. K., and J. Jerman, 2017. "Population Group Abortion Rates and Lifetime Incidence of Abortion: United States, 2008–2014." *American Journal of Public Health* 107 (12): 1904–9.

Jost, J. T., and A. C. Kay 2005. "Exposure to Benevolent Sexism and Complementary Gender Stereotypes: Consequences for Specific and Diffuse Forms of System Justification." *Journal of Personality and Social Psychology* 88 (3): 498–509.

Kaur, R., and S. Garg. 2008. "Addressing Domestic Violence Against Women: An Unfinished Agenda." *Indian Journal of Community Medicine* 33 (2): 73–76.

Kaye, K., J. A. Gootman, A. S. Ng, and C. Finley. 2014. *The Benefits of Birth Control in America: Getting the Facts Straight.* Washington, DC: The National Campaign to Prevent Teen and Unplanned Pregnancy. https://powertodecide.org/sites/default/files/resources/primary-download/benefits-of-birth-control-in -america.pdf.

Kerr, C. E., M. D. Sacchet, S. W. Lazar, C. I. Moore, and S. R. Jones. 2013. "Mindfulness Starts with the Body: Somatosensory Attention and Top-down Modulation of Cortical Alpha Rhythms in Mindfulness Meditation." *Frontiers in Human Neuroscience* 7: 12.

Kessler R. C., P. Berglund, O. Demler, R. Jin, K. R. Merikangas, and E. E. Walters. 2005. "Lifetime Prevalence and Age-of-Onset Distributions of DSM-IV Disorders in the National Comorbidity Survey Replication." *Archives of General Psychiatry* 62 (6): 593–602.

Klar, M., and T. Kasser. 2009. "Some Benefits of Being an Activist: Measuring Activism and Its Role in Psychological Well-Being." *Political Psychology* 30 (5): 755–77.

Ko, L. 2016. "Unwanted Sterilization and Eugenics Programs in the United States. Independent Lens." January 29. KQED *Independent Lens* (blog). http://www.pbs.org/independentlens/blog/unwanted-sterilization-and -eugenics-programs-in-the-united-states/

Krieger, N. 2005. "Embodiment: A Conceptual Glossary for Epistemology." *Journal of Epidemiology and Community Health* 59 (5): 350–55.

Kuehnel, S. S. 2009. "Abstinence-Only Education Fails African American Youth." *Washington University Law Review* 86 (5): 1241.

Lamont, J. M. 2015. "Trait Body Shame Predicts Health Outcomes in College Women: A Longitudinal Investigation." *Journal of Behavioral Medicine* 38 (6): 998–1008.

Landrine, H., and E. A. Klonoff, 1996. "The Schedule of Racist Events: A Measure of Racial Discrimination and a Study of Its Negative Physical and Mental Health Consequences." *Journal of Black Psychology* 22 (2): 144–68.

Lane, J., and J. W. Meeker. 2003. "Women's and Men's Fear of Gang Crimes: Sexual and Nonsexual Assault As Perceptually Contemporaneous Offenses." *Justice Quarterly* 20 (2): 337–71.

Lange, A. 2015. "14th and 15th Amendments." National Women's History Museum. Fall. http://www.crusade forthevote.org/14-15-amendments/.

Leighton, L. B. 2018. "The Trauma of Oppression: A Somatic Perspective." In *Oppression and the Body: Roots, Resistance, and Resolutions*, edited by C. Caldwell and L. B. Leighton. Berkeley, CA: North Atlantic Books.

Lilienfeld, S. O. 2017. "Microaggressions: Strong Claims, Inadequate Evidence." *Perspectives on Psychological Science* 12 (1): 138–69.

Lohman, B. J., T. K. Neppl, J. M. Senia, and T. J. Schofield. 2013. "Understanding Adolescent and Family Influences on Intimate Partner Psychological Violence During Emerging Adulthood and Adulthood." *Journal of Youth and Adolescence* 42 (4): 500–517.

Madestam, A., D. Shoag, S. Veuger, and D. Yanagizawa-Drott. 2013. "Do Political Protests Matter? Evidence from the Tea Party Movement." *Quarterly Journal of Economics* 128 (4): 1633–85.

Major, B., W. J., Quinton, and T. Schmader. 2003. "Attributions to Discrimination and Self-Esteem: Impact of Group Identification and Situational Ambiguity." *Journal of Experimental Social Psychology* 39 (3): 220–31.

Mann, T. 2015. *Secrets from the Eating Lab: The Science of Weight Loss, the Myth of Willpower and Why You Should Never Diet Again*. New York: Harper Collins.

Manne, K. 2018. *Down Girl: The Logic of Misogyny*. New York: Oxford University Press.

Mapping Police Violence. 2017. "2017 Police Violence Report." https://mappingpoliceviolence.org.

Mascarelli, A. L. 2015. "Explainer: Male-Female Flexibility in Animals." *Science News for Students*. July 31. https://www.sciencenewsforstudents.org/article/explainer-male-female-flexibility-animals.

Matos, K. 2015. *Modern Families: Same- and Different-Sex Couples Negotiating at Home*. New York: Families and Work Institute.

McCaig, A. 2018. "Psychologists: Women Are Not to Blame for the Wage Gap." *Rice University News and Media*. May 31. http://news.rice.edu/2018/05/31/psychologists-women-are-not-to-blame-for-the-wage-gap-2/.

McEwen, B. S. 2012. "Brain on Stress." *Proceedings of the National Academy of Sciences* 109 (Suppl 2): 17180–85.

McIntosh, P. 1989, 2010. "White Privilege: Unpacking the Invisible Knapsack." Wellesley Centers for Women. Excerpt from original 1989 paper. https://www.wcwonline.org/images/pdf/Knapsack_plus_Notes-Peggy _McIntosh.pdf.

McKinsey and Company. 2018. *Women in the Workplace 2018*. Lean In. https://womenintheworkplace .com/?mod=article_inline#pipeline-data.

McLean, C. P., A. Asnaani, B. T. Litz, and S. G. Hofmann. 2011. "Gender Differences in Anxiety Disorders: Prevalence, Course of Illness, Comorbidity, and Burden of Illness." *Journal of Psychiatric Research* 45 (8): 1027–35.

Möller, A., H. P. Söndergaard, and L. Helström. 2017. "Tonic Immobility During Sexual Assault: A Common Reaction Predicting Post-Traumatic Stress Disorder and Severe Depression." *Acta Obsetricia et Gynecologica Scandinavica* 96 (8): 932–38.

Montgomery, N., and C. Bergman. 2017. *Joyful Militancy: Building Thriving Resistance in Toxic Times*. Chico, CA: AK Press.

Moss, P., and A. Maddrell. 2017. "Emergent and Divergent Spaces in the Women's March: The Challenges of Intersectionality and Inclusion." *Gender, Place and Culture* 24 (5): 613–20.

Mustillo, S., N. Krieger, E. P. Gunderson, S. Sidney, H. McCreath and C. I. Kiefe, 2004. "Self-Reported. Experiences of Racial Discrimination and Black-White Differences in Preterm and Low-Birthweight Deliveries: The CARDIA Study." *American Journal of Public Health* 94 (12): 2125–31.

Namy, S., C. Carlson, K. O'Hara, J. Nakuti, P. Bukuluki, J. Lwanyaaga, S. Namakula, B. Nanyunja, M. L. Wainberg, D. Naker, and L. Michau. 2017. "Towards a Feminist Understanding of Intersecting Violence Against Women and Children in the Family." *Social Science and Medicine* 184: 40–48.

Natelson, R. 2017. "How Much Trash a Political Rally Leaves for Others to Clean Up Tells You Something, Doesn't It?" Independence Institute. March 6. https://i2i.org/how-much-trash-a-political-rally-leaves -for-others-to-clean-up-tells-you-something-doesnt-it/.

National Partnership for Women and Families. 2016. *By the Numbers: Women Continue to Face Pregnancy Discrimination in the Workplace: An Analysis of US Equal Employment Opportunity Commission Charges (Fiscal Years 2011–2015)*. Data brief. October. Washington, DC: National Partnership for Women and Families. http://www.nationalpartnership.org/research-library/workplace-fairness/pregnancy-discrimina-tion/by-the-numbers-women-continue-to-face-pregnancy-discrimination-in-the-workplace.pdf.

National Task Force on the Prevention and Treatment of Obesity. 2000. "Dieting and the Development of Eating Disorders in Overweight and Obese Adults." *Archives of Internal Medicine* 160 (17): 2581–90.

Nelson, J. 2015. *More Than Medicine: A History of the Feminist Women's Health Movement*. New York: NYU Press.

O'Brien, C. C. 2009. "'The White Women All Go for Sex': Frances Harper on Suffrage, Citizenship, and the Reconstruction South." *African American Review* 43 (4): 605–20.

Olds, T. 2016. "Your 'Ideal' Body, and Why You Want It." *The Conversation*. February 22. https://theconversa tion.com/your-ideal-body-and-why-you-want-it-53433.

Özascilar, M. 2013. "Predicting Fear of Crime: A Test of the Shadow of Sexual Assault Hypothesis." *International Review of Victimology* 19 (3): 269–84.

Paradis, E., A. Kuper, and R. K. Reznick. 2013. "Body Fat As Metaphor: From Harmful to Helpful." *Canadian Medical Association Journal* 185 (2): 152–53.

Parker, K., J. Menasce Horowitz, and R. Stepler. 2017. "On Gender Differences, No Consensus on Nature Vs. Nurture: Americans Say Society Places a Higher Premium on Masculinity Than on Femininity." Pew Research Center. December 5. http://www.pewsocialtrends.org/2017/12/05/on-gender-differences-no -consensus-on-nature-vs-nurture/.

Pearl, R. L., T. A. Wadden, C. M. Hopkins, J. A. Shaw, M. R. Hayes, Z. M. Bakizada, N. Alfaris, A. M. Chao, E. Pinkasavage, R. I. Berkowitz, and N. Alamuddin. 2017. "Association Between Weight Bias Internalization and Metabolic Syndrome Among Treatment-Seeking Individuals with Obesity." *Obesity (Silver Spring)* 25 (2): 317–22.

Peterson, R. D., S. Tantleff-Dunn, and J. S. Bedwell. 2006. "The Effects of Exposure to Feminist Ideology on Women's Body Image." *Body Image* 3 (3): 237–46.

Petrzela, N. M., and C. B. Whelan. 2018. "Self-Help Gurus Like Tony Robbins Have Often Stood in the Way of Social Change." *The Washington Post.* April 13. https://www.washingtonpost.com/outlook/self-help-gurus-like-tony-robbins-have-often-stood-in-the-way-of-social-change/2018/04/13/15340974-3e70-11e8-8d53-eba0ed2371cc_story.html?utm_term=.5a5819a25ddd.

Pew Research Center. 2018. "Public Opinion on Abortion: Views on Abortion, 1995-2018." Fact sheet. http://www.pewforum.org/fact-sheet/public-opinion-on-abortion/.

Pierce, C. 1970. "Offensive Mechanisms." In *The Black Seventies*, edited by F. L. Barbour. Boston: Porter Sargent.

Pinquart, M., and S. Sörensen. 2006. "Gender Differences in Caregiver Stressors, Social Resources, and Health: An Updated Meta-analysis." *The Journals of Gerontology: Series B, Psychological Sciences and Social Sciences* 61 (1): 33–45.

Pines, A. M. 1994. "Burnout in Political Activism: An Existential Perspective." *Journal of Health and Human Resources Administration* 16 (4): 381–94.

Phelan, J. E., D. T. Sanchez, and T. L. Broccoli, 2010. "The Danger in Sexism: The Links Among Fear of Crime, Benevolent Sexism, and Well-Being." *Sex Roles* 62 (1–2): 35–47.

Plyler, J. 2009. "How to Keep On Keeping On." *Upping the Anti* 3: 123–34.

Raymond, E. G., and D. A. Grimes. 2012. "The Comparative Safety of Legal Induced Abortion and Childbirth in the United States." *Obstetrics and Gynecology* 119 (2 Pt. 1): 215–19.

Reichert, J., and L. Bostwick. 2010. *Post-Traumatic Stress Disorder and Victimization Among Female Prisoners in Illinois.* A report for the Illinois Criminal Justice Information Authority. November. http://www.icjia.state.il.us/assets/pdf/ResearchReports/PTSD_Female_Prisoners_Report_1110.pdf.

Ross, L. 2017. "Reproductive Justice Beyond Biology." *Race and Ethnicity.* March 15. Center for American Progress. https://www.americanprogress.org/issues/race/news/2017/03/15/428191/reproductive-justice-beyond-biology/.

Ross, L. J., and R. Solinger. 2017. *Reproductive Justice: An Introduction.* Oakland, CA: University of California Press.

Schaufeli, W. B., and B. P. Buunk. 2002. "Burnout: An Overview of 25 Years of Research and Theorizing." In *The Handbook of Work and Health Psychology*, 2nd ed., edited by M. J. Schabracq, J. A. M. Winnubst, and C. L. Cooper. Chichester, UK: Wiley.

Schilt, K. 2006. "Just One of the Guys? How Transmen Make Gender Visible at Work." *Gender and Society* 20 (4): 465–90.

Schlafly, P., 1997. "G.I. Jane Is a Role-Model for Evil." *Eagle Forum.* September 10. http://eagleforum.org/column/1997/sept97/97-09-10.html.

Sechrist, G. B., and C. Delmar. 2009. "When Do Men and Women Make Attributions to Gender Discrimination? The Role of Discrimination Source." *Sex Roles* 61 (9): 607–20.

Shapiro, J., and J. Pupovac. 2008. "In Prison, Discipline Comes Down Hardest on Women." *All Things Considered.* October 15. https://www.npr.org/2018/10/15/647874342/in-prison-discipline-comes-down-hardest-on-womenthe

Smith, I. Z., K. L. Bentley-Edwards, S. El-Amin, and W. Darity, Jr. 2018. *Fighting at Birth: Eradicating the Black-White Infant Mortality Gap.* A report for the Samuel Dubois Cook Center of Social Equity and Insight Center for Community Economic Development at Duke University. March. https://socialequity.duke.edu/sites/socialequity.duke.edu/files/site-images/EradicatingBlackInfantMortality-March2018-DRAFT4.pdf.

Smith, S. G., J. Chen, K. C. Basile, L. K. Gilbert, M. T. Merrick, N. Patel, M. Walling, and A. Jain. 2017. *The National Intimate Partner and Sexual Violence Survey (NISVS): 2010-2012 State Report.* Atlanta, GA: National Center for Injury Prevention and Control, Centers for Disease Control and Prevention. https://www.cdc.gov/violenceprevention/pdf/NISVS-StateReportBook.pdf.

Stanger-Hall, K. F., and D. W. Hall. 2011. "Abstinence-Only Education and Teen Pregnancy Rates: Why We Need Comprehensive Sex Education in the US." *PLoS One* 6 (10): e24658.

Stein, P., S. Hendrix, and A. Hauslohner. 2017. "Women's Marches: More Than One Million Protesters Vow to Resist President Trump." *The Washington Post*, January 22. https://www.washingtonpost.com/local/womens-march-on-washington-a-sea-of-pink-hatted-protesters-vow-to-resist-donald-trump/2017/01/21/ae4def62-dfdf-11e6-acdf-14da832ae861_story.html?utm_term=.0b7faeb47c68.

Sue, D. W. 2010. "Microaggressions, Marginality, and Oppression: An Introduction." In *Microaggressions and Marginality: Manifestation, Dynamics and Impact*, edited by D.W. Sue. Hoboken, New Jersey: John Wiley and Sons.

Sue, D. W., C. M. Capodilupo, G. C. Torino, J. M. Bucceri, A. M. Holder, K. L. Nadal, and M. Esquilin. 2007. "Racial Microaggressions in Everyday Life: Implications for Clinical Practice." *The American Psychologist* 62 (4): 271–86.

Susmitha, B. 2016. "Domestic Violence: Causes, Impact and Remedial Measures." *Social Change* 46 (4): 602–10.

Swank, E., and B. Fahs. 2017. "Understanding Feminist Activism Among Women: Resources, Consciousness, and Social Networks." *Socius* 3.

Swim, J. K., L. L. Hyers, L. L. Cohen, and M. J. Ferguson, 2001. "Everyday Sexism: Evidence for Its Incidence, Nature, and Psychological Impact from Three Daily Diary Studies." *Journal of Social Issues* 57 (1): 31–53.

Sylaska, K. M., and K. M. Edwards. 2014. "Disclosure of Intimate Partner Violence to Informal Social Support Network Members: A Review of Literature." *Trauma, Violence, and Abuse* 15 (1): 3–21.

Symington, A. 2004. "Intersectionality: A Tool for Gender and Economic Justice, Facts, and Issues." The Association for Women's Rights in Development (AWID).

Tjaden, P., and N. Thoennes. 2000. "Full Report of the Prevalence, Incidence, and Consequences of Violence Against Women: Findings from the National Violence Against Women Survey." November. Washington, DC, and Atlanta, GA: National Institute of Justice and Centers for Disease Control and Prevention. https://www.ncjrs.gov/pdffiles1/nij/183781.pdf.

Veenstra, G. 2011. "Race, Gender, Class, and Sexual Orientation: Intersecting Axes of Inequality and Self-Rated Health in Canada." *International Journal for Equity in Health* 10: 3.

Walker, R. 1992. "Becoming the Third Wave." *Ms.* Magazine, January, 39–41.

Wang, T., D. Solomon, L. E., Durso, S. McBride, and S. Cahill. 2016. *State Anti-Transgender Bathroom Bills Threaten Transgender People's Health and Participation in Public Life.* Policy brief, Center for American Progress, the Fenway Institute. https://fenwayhealth.org/wp-content/uploads/2015/12/COM-2485-Transgender-Bathroom-Bill-Brief_v8-pages.pdf.

Webb, J., M. Fiery, and N. Jafari. 2016. "'You Better Not Leave Me Shaming!': Conditional Indirect Effect Analyses of Anti-Fat Attitudes, Body Shame, and Fat Talk As a Function of Self-Compassion in College Women." *Body Image* 18: 5–13.

Webster, S. H. 2017. "A Qualitative Study of the Evolution and Erasure of Black Feminism in Historic and Contemporary Sociopolitical Movements, and Black Men's Resistance to Black Feminism." *McNair Scholars Research Journal* 10 (1): Article 15.

Weldon, S. L., and M. Htun. 2013. "Feminist Mobilisation and Progressive Policy Change: Why Governments Take Action to Combat Violence Against Women." *Gender and Development* 21 (2): 231–47.

Wohlford, K. E., J. E. Lochman, and T. D. Barry. 2004. "The Relation Between Chosen Role Models and the Self-Esteem of Men and Women." *Sex Roles* 50 (7–8): 575–82.

Wong, K. 2018. "There's a Stress Gap between Men and Women. Here's Why It's Important." *The New York Times*, November 14. https://www.nytimes.com/2018/11/14/smarter-living/stress-gap-women-men.html.

World Health Organization. 2006. *Defining Sexual Health: Report of a Technical Consultation on Sexual Health*. Geneva: World Health Organization.

———. 2009. *Violence Prevention: The Evidence. Promoting Gender Equality to Prevent Violence Against Women*. Geneva: World Health Organization.

———. 2013. *Global and Regional Estimates of Violence Against Women: Prevalence and Health Effects of Intimate Partner Violence and Nonpartner Sexual*

Violence. Geneva: World Health Organization.

———. 2019. "Gender and Genetics." Genomic Resource Center. http://www.who.int/genomics/gender/en/index1.html.

Wyne, Z. 2015. "The Women Who Fought AIDS: 'It Was Never Not Our Battle.'" *Broadly*. August 28. https://broadly.vice.com/en_us/article/mbqjqp/the-women-who-fought-aids-it-was-never-not-our-battle.

Yavorsky, J. E., C. M. Dush, and S. J. Schoppe-Sullivan. 2015. "The Production of Inequality: The Gender Division of Labor Across the Transition to Parenthood." *Journal of Marriage and the Family* 77 (3): 662–79.

Yuan, N. P., M. P., Koss, and M. Stone. 2006. *The Psychological Consequences of Sexual Trauma*. March. Harrisburg, PA: National Online Resource Center on Violence Against Women. https://vawnet.org/material/psychological-consequences-sexual-trauma.

Zell, E., Z. Krizan, and S. R. Teeter. 2015. "Evaluating Gender Similarities and Differences Using Metasynthesis." *The American Psychologist* 70 (1): 10–20.

Zucker, A. N., and L. J. Landry. 2007. "Embodied Discrimination: The Relation of Sexism and Distress to Women's Drinking and Smoking Behaviors." *Sex Roles* 56 (3–4): 193–203.

Joanne L. Bagshaw, PhD, is an award-winning professor of psychology and women's studies at Montgomery College. She is also an ASSECT-certified sex therapist with a private practice in Maryland, where she lives with her husband and daughter. Joanne writes the popular feminist blog, *The Third Wave* for *Psychology Today*.

MORE BOOKS *from*
NEW HARBINGER PUBLICATIONS

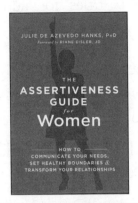

**THE ASSERTIVENESS GUIDE
FOR WOMEN**

How to Communicate Your Needs,
Set Healthy Boundaries &
Transform Your Relationships

978-1626253377 / US $16.95

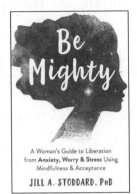

BE MIGHTY

A Woman's Guide to Liberation
from Anxiety, Worry & Stress Using
Mindfulness & Acceptance

978-1684034413 / US $16.95

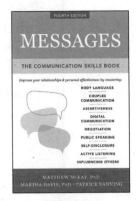

**MESSAGES,
FOURTH EDITION**

The Communications
Skills Book

978-1684031719 / US $21.95

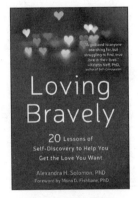

LOVING BRAVELY

Twenty Lessons of
Self-Discovery to Help You
Get the Love You Want

978-1626255814 / $16.95

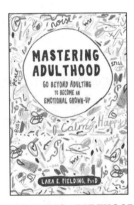

MASTERING ADULTHOOD

Go Beyond Adulting to Become
an Emotional Grown-Up

978-1684031931 / US $16.95

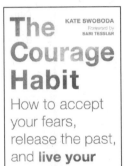

THE COURAGE HABIT

How to Accept Your Fears, Release
the Past & Live Your Courageous Life

978-1626259874 / US $17.95

newharbingerpublications
1-800-748-6273 / newharbinger.com

(VISA, MC, AMEX / prices subject to change without notice)

Follow Us [f] [t] [i] [p]

Don't miss out on new books in the subjects that interest you.
Sign up for our **Book Alerts** at **newharbinger.com/bookalerts**

Register your **new harbinger** titles for additional benefits!

When you register your **new harbinger** title—purchased in any format, from any source—you get access to benefits like the following:

- Downloadable accessories like printable worksheets and extra content
- Instructional videos and audio files
- Information about updates, corrections, and new editions

Not every title has accessories, but we're adding new material all the time.

Access free accessories in 3 easy steps:

1. Sign in at NewHarbinger.com (or **register** to create an account).

2. Click on **register a book**. Search for your title and click the **register** button when it appears.

3. Click on the **book cover or title** to go to its details page. Click on **accessories** to view and access files.

That's all there is to it!

If you need help, visit:

NewHarbinger.com/accessories

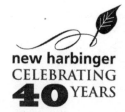

new harbinger
CELEBRATING
40 YEARS